DEAFENED PEOPLE:
ADJUSTMENT AND SUPPORT

D0752717

It is estimated that there are currently 1.9 million deafened people living in North America – individuals who could once hear naturally or
with amplification but have become deaf and are now unable to rely
on hearing to comprehend spoken information. Despite this vast number, until now there have been few books that specifically address the
process of adjustment to, and acceptance of, deafness as an adult.
Kathryn Woodcock and Miguel Aguayo have addressed that situation
with their unique look at deafness in *Deafened People: Adjustment and
Support*.

The authors demonstrate that deafness is not merely a medical condition; it is a social disability that affects the individual, the family, the
social circle, and the work group. By describing the psychosocial experience of acquired deafness as a process of adjustment, Woodcock and
Aguayo demonstrate that acceptance of deafness is a process with
practical, social, and emotional implications. To assist in that process,
the authors have provided a guide to self-help techniques of proven
value to deafened people.

Drawing on their own experiences as deaf professionals, Woodcock
and Aguayo explore such questions as how deafness occurs, how relationships (professional and personal) can be affected by progressive
deafness, and how and where to find peer support. Section 1 describes
the process of adjustment, while Section 2 offers a practical guide to a
successful method of establishing a self-help support network, with
reference to such organizations as the Association of Late-Deafened
Adults. Written in a lively, engaging style, the book combines medical
background, professional advice, information on resources, and personal examples. *Deafened People: Adjustment and Support* will be invalu-
able for medical professionals and lay readers alike.

KATHRYN WOODCOCK is Associate Professor in the School of Occupational and Public Health at Ryerson Polytechnic University.

MIGUEL AGUAYO is a registered social worker specializing in deafness –
particularly acquired deafness – and other disabilities. A consultant to
social service agencies on information technology and organizational
change, he is currently a coordinator for the Ontario March of Dimes.

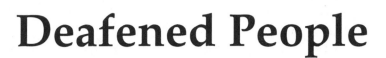

Deafened People

Adjustment and Support

KATHRYN WOODCOCK
MIGUEL AGUAYO

UNIVERSITY OF TORONTO PRESS
Toronto Buffalo London

ISBN 0-8020-4845-5 (cloth)
ISBN 0-8020-8373-0 (paper)

Printed on acid-free paper

Canadian Cataloguing in Publication Data

Woodcock, Kathryn Lee, 1956–
    Deafened people : adjustment and support

    Includes bibliographical references and index.
    ISBN 0-8020-4845-5 (bound)   ISBN 0-8020-8373-0 (pbk.)

    1. Deaf.   2. Postlingual deafness.   3. Deaf – Services for.
    4. Self-help techniques.   I. Aguayo, Miguel Oswald.   II. Title.

    HV2380.W66 2000   362.4'2   C00-931736-8

The University of Toronto Press acknowledges the financial assistance
to its publishing program of the Canada Council for the Arts and the
Ontario Arts Council.

University of Toronto Press acknowledges the financial support for its
publishing activities of the Government of Canada through the Book
Publishing Industry Development Program (BPIDP).

To Ruby

Contents

viii   Contents

Preface

This book about deafened adults discusses acquired deafness (adventitious deafness, late deafness) from a new perspective: adjustment. Other books have described how deafness disrupts and perhaps even devastates the lives of adults who acquire the condition, but few have discussed the lengthy process of adjustment except in the form of biographies – and biographies, by their nature, are about people who are exceptional rather than typical. Yes, acquired deafness hinders relationships. Yes, those who acquire deafness are caught between the hearing and deaf worlds. Yet somehow, most people survive. The struggle, protracted and arduous though it may be, eventually resolves itself in some degree of adjustment. That adjustment might be easier, and perhaps a little more successful, if more guidance was available for deafened adults and for professionals. While we think our contribution makes a good start, we hope to see more research into specific supports for improved emotional adjustment. Till now, there has been too narrow an emphasis on the vocational adaptation and aural rehabilitation of this population.

In this book, we describe acquired deafness and its impact, and present our model of the adjustment process. We then outline different sources of help: professional help, peer help, and the most important – self-help. Although self-help has been a cornerstone of deafened adults' associations, there has not been a printed reference that deafened adults can consult to learn how to set up self-help support groups. The peer help and self-help chapters are written specifically for deafened people who are interested in organizing and leading self-help groups for deafened adults. We hope this book will be a useful introduction and guide to acquired deafness and a resource that professionals can recommend to deafened clients.

The first four chapters describe the impact of acquired deafness on the deafened person and relationships. They focus on *adjustment* and are written from a professional orientation. We hope that deafened people will find them a source of personal insight. Even more, we hope these chapters will provide insight for professionals who work with deafened clients. The remaining chapters are written for our fellow deafened people who are interested in providing support and accessing self-help. We hope professionals will find them useful to pass along to clients who are interested, and ready to heal and grow.

We have designed this book to present both objective and subjective information on this topic. As deafened people, we offer our experiences and comments in boxes within the text. We hope that professionals will recognize that our own experiences validate the issues we raise.

For the Deafened Reader

You need to understand that although we are deafened – perhaps like you – we don't know what is best for you. Neither does anybody else. The only person who can ever know what is best for you is you. All the laws and skills and technical 'facts' you will encounter are based on what was best for somebody else.

There are few references that deafened people can use to help them understand their particular situation. There are plenty of books on the market about deaf culture issues, and about living with milder hearing losses than we have, but we need books about *us*. We need books that talk about how many of us there are, and what we have gone through in becoming deaf, and how to organize and run self-help in our communities. Finally, we need books we can tell our professionals to read. This book provides information on becoming deaf that professionals can learn from, and that perhaps deafened people can also learn from, as well as detailed information on organizing and leading self-help groups for deafened adults. It complements out Internet website 'The Deafened People Page' (www.deafened.org), where supplementary information can be found. We hope this book will help deafened people *help* themselves adjust to deafness so that they can get back to *being* themselves!

We will assume that the reader is familiar with the names of technical devices such as TTY and captioning, and with deafness-related terms, although we provide some background on these topics.

To avoid resorting to 'them' as a genderless singular pronoun, we have used *him* and *her* randomly throughout the book. We can think of no case where changing the gender would compel us to change any of our propositions.

About the Authors

Dr Kathryn Woodcock deafened progressively through her teenage and twenties. She is an ergonomist by training and earned degrees in human factors engineering/-ergonomics from the University of Waterloo and the University of Toronto. Her research has incorporated deafness, hearing loss, and reasonable accommodation issues, but her principal research pertains to occupational safety: accident analysis, safety measurement, and qualitative methodologies. She is presently Associate Professor in the School of Occupational and Public Health at Ryerson Polytechnic University. Dr Woodcock is also a consultant to several research and social service organizations. She previously taught engineering and ergonomics at both the University of Waterloo and the Rochester Institute of Technology. For eight years before beginning her doctoral studies, she was Vice President, Hospital Services, at Centenary Health Centre in Toronto. Prior to that, she held positions in business, industry, and research. Dr Woodcock has been active in community service, and is a recipient of the Professional Engineers Ontario Community Service Medal, the Canadian Council of Professional Engineers Medal for Distinguished Achievement, and the Ontario Medal of Good Citizenship – Ontario's highest award for voluntarism. She presently serves on the board of governors of Centennial College in Toronto, and on the Advisory Board of the National Captioning Institute. She has served in various capacities on many other bodies, including the Ontario Council of Regents, the Advisory Committee on Hearing Aid Services, the board of directors of the National Captioning Institute, the Canadian Standards Association technical advisory committee on work injury statistics, and the Executive Council of the Human Factors Association of Canada. She was co-founder of the Canadian Deafened Persons Association, director and secretary of the Association of Late-Deafened Adults, and the first deaf president of the board of the Canadian Hearing Society. She has received numerous other awards for her achievements, including the Lyons Memorial Lectureship at the National Technical Institute for the Deaf, the Outstanding Alumni Award for the University of Waterloo Faculty of Engineering, the International Alumni of Delta Epsilon Sorority award for deaf women doctoral candidates, and the First Deaf Achievers award from the Ontario Association of the Deaf. Dr Woodcock is the webmaster of The Deafened People Page on the World Wide Web, and founder and three times editor of the Association of Late-Deafened Adults *Reader*, an annual anthology. She has published numerous articles on both ergonomics and late deafness.

Miguel Aguayo is a social worker who became deaf suddenly due to meningitis while in his teens. His hearing fluctuated for several years but then deteriorated completely. Twenty years after becoming deaf, he received one of the earliest 22-channel cochlear implants. He received his baccalaureate degree in social work from Rochester Institute of Technology, where he won the Outstanding Baccalaureate Student Award from the National Technical Institute for the Deaf. He earned a Master of Social Work degree at Wilfrid Laurier University; while there, he conducted thesis research into the effectiveness of rehabilitation services for deafened adults. He has spoken about social work and deafened adults and about cochlear implants to various audiences, and also written on those subjects. Mr Aguayo is presently working as a coordinator for Ontario March of Dimes. He has also consulted to social service organizations on both information technology and organizational change. He is a Registered Social Worker and holds additional certificates in mediation, use of the Myers-Briggs Type Indicator, human sexuality counselling, and self-help leadership. He is presently co-chair and dispute resolution panelist for the Ministry of Community and Social Services Ontario Disability Support Program (Toronto region), and a Director of Silent Voice, a social service agency for the deaf. Mr Aguayo was a member of the original Chicago ALDA self-help group and served as one of its leaders for three years, as well as several terms on the board of the Chicago chapter, and was elected to the ALDA board of directors. He co-founded the Recovery special interest group in ALDA and has led Recovery/Friends of Bill W. self-help and lecture/ workshop sessions at ALDA conventions. He is also a 3rd Dan black belt in Tae Kwon Do, and competed in regional level tournaments until he was medically disqualified from competition due to his cochlear implant.

PART ONE

Adjustment

Chapter 1

About Late Deafness

Although it has been over twenty years since the last major census of the deaf, the best estimate we have is that 75 per cent of deaf adults became deaf after the age of nineteen.[1] Most people in the deaf community probably don't think of late-deafened people as the majority. Services provided to 'the deaf' are directed overwhelmingly at people who became deaf at birth or in early childhood. Funding and subsidies for 'deaf' organizations go overwhelmingly to that segment. When you think of access to services for 'deaf' people, you think of sign language interpreting. And you think of sign language as being the native language of the deaf population. Yet the majority of deaf people acquired their condition later in childhood, in young adulthood, during their working years, or later in life.

When people think of adults becoming deaf, they typically think of Granny losing her hearing and being shouted at during the family reunion. Actually this image is of a hard-of-hearing person rather than of a deafened person. Many people do become hard of hearing due to normal aging processes, overexposure to noise, and other causes. That being said, there's a big difference between being hard of hearing and becoming deaf.

It has been asserted that deafened people first experience being hard of hearing. The implication is that deafness is the extreme case of hard of hearing and that the coping techniques and needs of both are therefore the same and have already been acquired. Actually, the majority of deafened people go from hearing to deaf with little opportunity to prepare.

1.1 Hearing and Hearing Loss

We will not expand on the science of the sense of hearing because we do not want to distract readers from our main theme, which is emotional and practical adjustment. However, it is worth clarifying some basic concepts.

1.1.1 What Does the Audiogram Have to Do with Speech Communication?

Hearing loss is measured on an audiogram chart, or sometimes a table with a list of numbers. The list of numbers is used to reduce the writing space required, or to document hearing loss over time. The professionals mentally or physically plot the numbers on an audiogram graph.

The vertical lines on the chart represent the frequency measured in hertz (Hz), which used to be called cycles per second (cps) and still means the same thing. Musicians use the term 'pitch' for roughly (but not exactly) the same concept as frequency. The increment between the equally spaced lines is a doubling of frequency: 500 Hz is exactly the same distance from 250 Hz as it is from 1000 Hz (or 1 kHz, as it is sometimes written). The scale along the bottom typically goes from 250 or 500 Hz up to 4000 or 8000 Hz (4 kHz or 8 kHz). Middle C on the piano is 256 Hz. Human speech falls mainly in the range of 300–3000 Hz, except for a few little sounds, such as the /th/ sound in 'thin,' which has components up in the 6000 Hz range. The 'banana' shape on Figure 1.1 corresponds roughly to where speech sounds are. The horizontal lines indicate how loud[2] the sound has to be before you hear it. That explains why the scale on the left side goes from 0 at the top down to 100 or 110 decibels (dB) at the bottom, which is the reverse of how graphs are usually constructed. The result is that the graph of your hearing will be low where you have low hearing (i.e., a hearing loss), and

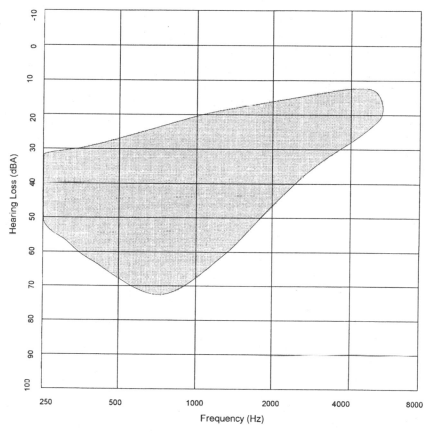

Figure 1.1: Audiogram, Speech Range, and Hearing Loss

high where you have good hearing. Actually, there is the possibility of a negative measurement, so the scale often goes to –10 above the zero line at the top. The reason is that decibels are a ratio of a particular sound to some standard-loudness sound (the 'ANSI' standard). Zero decibels is the loudness of a sound that 'normal' human hearing can just barely detect. This is similar to the measurement of your eyesight compared to 20/20. People with sharper vision get a measurement of 20/15 or 20/10, while those who need glasses score 20/40 or worse. If you can hear a particular frequency at a softer level than that standard loudness sound, then good for you – you have a negative decibel reading for that tone: better than normal hearing. Note that a price increase from $50 to $60 is a 20 per cent rise, but an increase from 50 to 60 decibels isn't 20 per cent louder. Because the decibel scale is logarithmic, an increase of 10 decibels is 10 *times* as intense.[3]

To measure hearing and plot the audiogram, the audiologist plays tones of different frequency and loudness through a headset, and also through the bone behind the ear. (Old-fashioned screening may involve a piano-tuning fork held near the ear, and/or placed on the skull.) The tones are played with background noise in the other ear and under other assorted conditions. The objective is to find the quietest sound level that can just barely be heard: the hearing threshold. On hearing the sound, the patient will raise a hand or press a button, and the audiologist will record the level and adjust to the next sound level or frequency. The quietest audible level measured for each frequency through the headset is the 'air conduction' threshold; the quietest level through the bone headband is the 'bone conduction' threshold. Full audiometry usually also involves repeating one-syllable and two-syllable words so that the percentage heard correctly can be recorded. 'Comfortable loudness' is measured as well; some people find louder sounds more uncomfortable. Sensitivity to loud sound can result in a very narrow window between just loud enough and way too loud. A full hearing test takes about an hour, usually in a little soundproof booth.

1.1.2 *So How Much of a Hearing Loss Is That?*

Hearing loss is hard to describe, and resorting to dimensions of the sort we use to describe our eyesight, fitness, or IQ is no solution. There is no such thing as a 'percentage' hearing loss. Even descriptions of 'x decibel' hearing loss are meaningless unless you indicate which frequencies the loss affects. Some people have a more or less equal decibel hearing loss across all frequencies. Others have a big loss at some frequencies and a milder loss at others. The important thing is the amount of hearing loss in the speech range. One way to indicate this is by averaging the decibel loss at 500, 1000, and 2000 Hz, but even this only provides an indication. A person with a 70 dB loss at each of these frequencies will hear a different version of the world than someone who has a 30 dB loss at 500, an 80 dB loss at 1000, and a 100 dB loss at 2000 Hz, which averages 70 dB. The kinds of hearing aids prescribed to these two people can vary widely, and so can the effectiveness of those hearing aids. No one should presume to understand what another person can hear and not hear based only on a single-number indicator of his or her hearing level.

Most people understand that deafness is not equivalent to silence. People may be deaf yet still be able to hear sounds. What makes deafness what it is, is the loss of ability to comprehend speech. Hearing environmental sounds – fire truck sirens, orchestral music, the ominous approach of footsteps in the dark – is an asset. However, it is the ability to communicate easily using spoken language that separates people we consider hearing from people we consider deaf. If a person somehow lost the ability to hear every sound *except* speech, we would consider her unfortunate, but probably not *deaf*, and perhaps not even disabled. In sum, it is the impact of hearing loss on speech that we must discuss.

Once you understand just what it is people need to understand speech, you will understand more about what audiograms say about which sounds are heard and which are missed.

1.1.3 How Does Loss of a Few Sounds Affect Speech?

Speech is made up of *phonemes*. Phonemes are the building blocks of language: more or less, they are 'letter-sounds.' They do not really depend on the alphabet, although we have to use some kind of alphabet to write them down. Every language has its own set of phonemes, even languages that use the same alphabet. Trying to say words like *merci* (the French *r* sound) or Loch Ness (the throaty *ch* sound) gives some English speakers difficulty because to them, these words contain alien phonemes.

English consists of forty-eight phonemes (Hawaiian has only eleven).[4] Only sixty phonemes are required to describe the speech sounds made in all the languages in the world.

Each phoneme takes only a brief slice of time before another phoneme comes along. Now imagine that you have recorded the speech signal. By feeding that signal through a computer, you can analyse the sound energy of each phoneme separately, and even graph that energy against the time axis.[5] Each phoneme consists of sound energy in a specific frequency combination. These combinations are quite consistent from person to person.[6] Consonants are either voiced (like the sounds we make for *b*, *d*, and *z*) or unvoiced (like the sounds of *p*, *t*, and *s*). Consonants classified as *fricatives* (the sounds of *f*, *v*, *th*, *s*, and *sh*, and the like) contribute a burst of irregularly shaped energy that looks like television static. Vowels have two or three dominant frequency bands in their sound energy, called *formants*. (Voiced consonants may also have one formant, or 'voice bar,' that reflects the frequency of the voicing.) Graphed along the time axis, the steady horizontal (same-frequency) bars of the vowel in the spectrogram may be preceded and/or followed by a rise or fall of the frequency, depending on the consonants on either side of the vowel. Consonants are discriminated from the transitions of vowels (as the rise or fall of one or more vowel formants, or as a stop gap when there is no sound energy at all), and from the presence or absence of the voice sound. The transitions – especially the transition in the vowel's second formant (the higher-frequency one) – and the onset and delay of voicing and fricative sounds help us identify which consonant was spoken.

Telling the phonemes apart requires hearing the frequency spectrum of sound energy, voicing, and transition cues. If background noise is loud, it may be hard to identify whether a phoneme was voiced or voiceless. If hearing is damaged only in a certain frequency range, some phonemes may be only partially affected. Unfortunately, the portion that is not heard may be the one that makes two phonemes sound different, and this is where speech sounds start to sound alike, for example, /f/ and /s/. It is also the reason why a person may be unable to understand speech, even though he swears that he can hear and that everything sounds just as loud as before.

1.2 How People Are Deafened

Understanding the *amount* of hearing loss goes only part of the way to answering other key questions: What effect does the hearing loss have? How deaf is this person? What should he (or I) be able to accomplish with (or in spite of) this particular loss? This is where the classification of hearing losses can be useful.

Oversimplified Anatomy and Physiology of the Ear

Figure 1.2 provides an illustration of the outer, middle, and inner ear.

   Outer ear: The big thing on the side of your head, and the ear canal, which you should never stick anything smaller than your elbow into, because at the inner end of it is the eardrum, which is delicate.
   Middle ear: A cavity inside the temporal bone, in which you will find little bones with the nicknames *hammer, anvil*, and *stirrup*. These are held in place by muscles and ligaments. The middle ear is full of air. There is a tube (the Eustachian tube) from this cavity to your throat that helps equalize the pressure around the eardrum – for example, when your airplane takes off.
   Inner ear: A fluid-filled section with two components. The *semicircular canals* handle the balance function, and the snail-shaped *cochlea* contains the nerve for hearing. Little hair cells line the cochlea – 16,000 of them, lined up in rows – ready to transform the mechanical vibrations of sound into nerve impulses, by way of the eighth cranial nerve.
   When a sound occurs, the pressure waves in the air travel through the ear canal and cause the eardrum to vibrate like,

well, a drum. Like the gears of a machine, the little bones on the other side of the eardrum transfer the vibration to the opening of the inner ear. This causes the inner-ear fluid to slosh around in time with those vibrations, causing the hair cells to sway like a field of wheat in the wind. The movement of the hair cells is relayed to the auditory nerves.

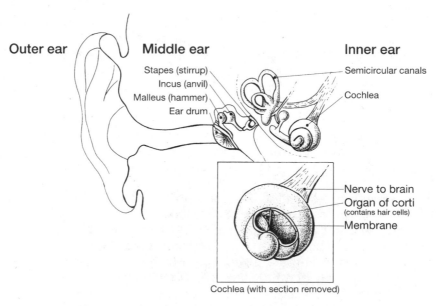

Figure 1.2: A look into the ear. Illustration courtesy of Monique LeBlanc.

1.2.1 Medical Classification of Hearing Loss

Medical professionals classify hearing loss as *conductive, senso-rineural*, or *mixed*. (Less commonly used are central and functional losses.) Doctors use these classifications to figure out and describe where the apparatus doesn't work, and determine whether they can make it work. Following is a simple summary of the main three categories.[7]

Conductive losses are failures in the middle ear, the outer ear, the Eustachian tubes, or the little windows. With conductive losses, the audiogram tends to be flattish or sloping upwards (showing better hearing) in the higher frequencies, and the loss is usually not more than 70 dB. These indicators, along with other ones such as a reduction only in air conduction (i.e., you can hear better if the sound is input directly to your skull or teeth), allow the doctor to identify a conductive hearing loss. People with conductive losses do not tend to have problems discriminating speech: if they can hear it, they can understand it. These people may be hard for *others* to hear, as they speak quieter and quieter. This is because their own voices – heard through the bone – sound much louder to them than others', which they hear through air alone.

A conductive loss is often happy news, because the prognosis is often good. A fairly flat audiogram doesn't prevent people from understanding speech that is loud enough, and a loss of even 70 dB makes amplification (i.e., hearing aids) quite feasible. As well, many conductive losses are caused by conditions that can be put right or at least relieved – for example, otosclerosis, or a perforated eardrum, or wax accumulation, or even a foreign object. A severe conductive hearing loss, or even a moderate one, can disrupt communication; even so, a purely conductive loss, if fully treated, permits a person to consider herself hard of hearing rather than deafened.

Sensorineural losses are failures in the inner ear, including the cochlea (sensory loss), or in the auditory nerve (the latter is a neural or 'retrocochlear' loss, often referred to as 'nerve deafness'). Both sensory and neural components may be present, or it may not be possible to rule out one or the other, and often it may simply not matter – hence the term 'sensorineural.'

If substantial damage occurs to the hair cells lining the cochlea, the nerve degenerates. The hair cells in the cochlea are in inner and outer groups. Almost all of the auditory nerve fibres go to the inner hair cells. Although the outer hair cells have few nerve connections, hearing loss occurs when they are damaged. The frequency range affected by the loss will be directly related to the location of the damaged area. That is, poor hearing will correspond to the damaged hair cells; other frequencies will be unaffected. If the hearing loss is somewhere in the middle frequency range only, the audiogram will have a notch or a dip. Often, we see damage in the high frequencies (i.e., we see a line that is horizontal on the left but sloping down on the right). A low-frequency loss is less common, and looks the opposite (i.e., low on the left and sloping up to the right).

Head trauma and noise tend to deteriorate the outer hair cells starting with the outer row; ototoxic medications tend to deteriorate them from the inner row. If the damage is only to the outer hairs, the loss will be 50 dB or less; for greater loss, there needs to be inner hair cell damage also. Other cochlear failures are possible, such as diminished movement of the cochlear partition, or damage in the nerve itself. For those who are not physicians, this is really all just a curiosity; there's nothing much the deafened person can do with this information.

Because the hearing loss may be pronounced at some frequencies and negligible at others, speech discrimination is a major problem. Even when someone's voice sounds loud, it may be completely unintelligible.

The prognosis for sensorineural loss is poor. Although *some* cases clear up, and *some* improvements can be achieved with therapy, 'it behooves the physician to tell the patient in a forthright manner that recovery of hearing is unlikely.'[8] The physician will probably next proceed to determine whether the loss is likely to be progressive.

Mixed hearing losses include some conductive and some sensory or neural damage. The damage may have occurred at the same time (e.g., with head injury) or at different times – for example, through diseases, or through injury and a disease, or through side effects from the treatment of the original hearing loss. An example of the latter: the surgery to fix otosclerosis, which is a conductive loss, can lead to an infection that causes sensorineural damage to the inner ear. The physician will be more enthusiastic about treatment if there is more conductive loss, as opposed to just a little bit of conductive but mostly sensorineural. For example, when a person with a very severe sensorineural loss punctures an eardrum or develops some wax buildup (conductive loss), fixing these will not repair the sensorineural component. The physician must determine how much of each component is there and then arrive at an appropriate treatment.

These classifications support the physician's role, which is centred on making a prognosis and proceeding from there to arrive at a medical therapy. The various tests used to make these classifications involve exploring the entire hearing system to isolate the location or locations of the damage. Having done that, the specialist can determine whether the damage can be repaired.

Generally, we find that this talk of sensorineural versus conductive is not very helpful for *deafened* people, except that it gives a name to what has happened. Most of the time, 'You have sensorineural hearing loss' is useful for about the length of time it takes to walk to the doctor's parking lot. As helpful as it is to the physician and to other professionals, and as essential as it is for determining what treatment, if any, is practical, that information does not tell the person *why* it happened. And even if the reason is, 'You were hit on the head and all the bones in your inner ear crumbled to dust,' it doesn't explain *why* you were hit on the head, and *why* you went out that day. The deafened person needs an explanation for why *she* doesn't hear, not why *her ears* don't hear. Her question is, *Why me? Why now? Why deafness and not some other way to build character?*

Perhaps it is really *these* questions that underlie the quest for a diagnosis. Yet even the most detailed diagnosis doesn't help the individual evaluate his feelings about his condition – in particular, how normal those feelings are. In this area, medical diagnosis can provide little help. The most useful response to the deafened person's question is to reverse it and ask, 'Why *not* you?' This brings us to the Experiential Classification of Acquired Deafness, not as a substitute for the medical diagnosis required for medical evaluation, but as a framework for social rehabilitation and individual adjustment.

1.3 Experiential Classification of Acquired Deafness

Our classification focuses on the felt experience of deafened people and recognizes the *changes* involved in becoming deaf. We extracted a classification structure from the stories of hundreds of deafened friends and acquaintances. Among these stories, there seem to be four broad etiologies of hearing loss: *medical, surgical, traumatic,* and *progressive*. (A fifth category, *psychiatric*, is rare but worth mentioning.) In the years since we first proposed this classification,[9] people informally have given it positive feedback. Unlike the classifications 'conductive' and 'sensorineural,' they seem to be able to grasp it instinctively, and to find it helpful for understanding the similarities and differences of their experiences. It is worth noting that most deafened people have sensorineural losses of different types, or mixed losses that include some sensorineural loss. To a physician, their prognosis may be the same; but their *experiences* vary, and those variations are meaningful as a point of orientation. That these experiential classes have inherent meaning for deafened people is indicated by the fact that categories such as these have been used in surveys that deafened people have conducted among themselves. See, for example, the surveys made by the National Association of Deafened People (U.K.) and the Association of Late-Deafened Adults (Figure 1.3 provides examples).

It may seem strange that we are suggesting that categories based on the location of auditory damage and on prognosis are not helpful to deafened people, but that experiential categories are. Surely, different experiences are encountered within each experiential group: for example, differences between overnight medical losses and gradual medical losses, and between progressive loss in adolescence and progressive loss in late adulthood. Yet experiential classifications are the ones that groups for deafened people reach for instinctively when conducting their own membership analyses.

The experiential classification is not predictive: membership in a particular category does not predetermine that a particular approach will work. How, then, can it help? Our observation is that this classification framework reassures people that their own experience need not match some other person's, or their own expectations. People who are not deaf (or who were not deaf before, but have become deaf) tend to regard deafness rather homogeneously. Exposure to the experiential classification helps them see that different experiences can explain their different reactions, different coping techniques, and different successes. Rather than forcing people to expect identical experiences within their 'class,' the framework invites them to seek greater *nuances*, and to start talking about deafness in terms of its variety.

1.3.1 Medical

Medical hearing losses are those resulting from chronic or acute illnesses such as Menière's syndrome; other syndromes, diseases, and infections; reactions to ototoxic medications; and 'The Virus.' A friend of ours (a Virus guy himself) likes to say, 'Whenever doctors don't know what something is, it's a virus.' It is comforting to disparage the authority that hasn't fixed the unfixable. Actually, these viruses include cytomegalovirus, the mumps, rubeola, chicken pox, influenza, adenovirus, and

Epstein-Barr. For all the difference it makes, it's just as well not to dwell on which.

Some people with medical losses become deaf overnight; others become deaf more gradually, say, over five or ten years. But even that is not as slow as the typical progressive-loss case. The onset of a medical hearing loss can usually be linked to some illness. Many of our acquaintances lost their hearing as a result of an illness so severe that, at the time, deafness was the least of their problems. They tell of their deafness being given short shrift by caregivers who, because of the training they had, were more adept at dealing with the illness itself than with the deafness it caused. Those with multiple medical problems often complain that both caregivers and family deal less well with their deafness than with any of their other conditions.

Sudden hearing loss often receives a highly 'medicalized' response, as the patient and doctors try various therapies (although there is no treatment available that is widely accepted as being better than 'wait and see'). A sudden loss rarely returns to normal when the other ear already has abnormal hearing. The likelihood that hearing will be restored is lower the more severe the loss and the more vertigo (dizziness) there is. Also, people younger than fifteen and older than sixty are less likely to recover from sudden hearing loss.[10]

Medical losses may not be profound, and it is not uncommon for medically deafened people to have conflicts with professionals and others who believe they should be able to function as well as a person with the same amount of residual hearing who has always been hard of hearing. Too often it is forgotten that a lack of experience at lipreading, and at coping generally, may render the residual hearing functionally useless. The perceived marked contrast with one's former hearing makes it easy for recently deafened people to accept that they need to acquire deaf tools: a caption decoder, TTY, and so on.

Some medical conditions, such as Menière's syndrome, come with other symptoms besides hearing loss, such as dizziness. This interferes even further with the normal activities of daily life, such as walking, working, and driving.

1.3.2 Surgical

Usually, people with surgical hearing loss knew when they went in for surgery that they would be deaf when they came out. Typically, their surgery was necessary in order to remove tumours on the auditory nerves: neurofibromatosis type-2 (NF-2) and bilateral acoustic neuromas. Forewarned does not necessarily mean forearmed, either for the patient or for the hospital. We have found that even with the luxury of advance warning, there is rarely any preparation or counselling available for these people. (In our view, a clinic that does this sort of surgery should have a qualified transcriptionist standing by to help the patient communicate during post-operative care. This is no different from hospitals having sign language interpreters available for deaf patients.)

Severing the auditory nerve creates an absolutely silent world (which may not be as annoying as dealing with people who persist in providing information on new hearing aids they just read about in the paper). Amplification and cochlear implants have nothing to offer a severed auditory nerve. Perhaps brainstem implants might work, or perhaps they might turn out to work for some but not for others (further complicating interactions with well-meaning strangers bearing advice).

Besides causing deafness, NF-2 requires patients to undergo multiple operations. Often these people sustain facial paralysis on one side. This may interfere with the clarity of their speech, and make it hard for other deaf people to lipread them.

1.3.3 Traumatic

Traumatic losses are incurred in a wide variety of exciting and adventurous ways, from motorcycle riding to settling an argument in an alley behind a bar. Many people confronting traumatic loss of hearing complain that professionals resort too quickly to the 'you're lucky to be alive' argument. Also, professionals may consider it premature to deal with a trauma victim's sudden deafness: the deafness may well be temporary. Even so, it would probably be easier for the patient to cope with surprise at getting her hearing back than with the dashing of false hopes. While deafness may not be the most urgent problem a trauma victim faces, once she has stabilized, it quickly becomes a matter of urgency – being bedridden and on painkillers leaves little to do except talk to visitors. Finally, new deafness can easily complicate the long-term treatment for any other concurrent injuries, since it interferes with communication with therapists and caregivers.

When the other injuries have healed and the deafness persists, some people (employers, insurers, family) may insinuate that the deafness is not genuine. Deafness from traumatic causes can be overlaid with lots of 'if only's': 'If only I hadn't been there ...' 'If only I had taken a cab ...' The anniversary of the event can revive the sense of loss.

1.3.4 Progressive

Some progressive losses result from aging – though simple presbycusis is usually a milder loss – and from exposure to excessive noise. Most noise cases seem to be mild or moderate; severe losses are in the minority. However, as common as noise-induced hearing loss is, this minority is still a substantial number. Some deafened adults had a previously mild medical hearing loss that was pushed over the brink into deafness by occupational noise exposure.

There is a form of hereditary hearing loss that is progressive. There is also an idiopathic form (i.e., one with no known cause). Medical losses can also occur gradually, but they usually have a known point of onset and result in deterioration over five to ten years, wreaking havoc along the way with the other symptoms of the illness. In contrast, progressive losses tend to sneak up over as many as twenty or thirty years, and can become quite severe before being detected.

If we may generalize a bit about rates of progression, many progressive losses of the hereditary or idiopathic type are mild or moderate by the teen years, and become severe to profound by the twenties and thirties, though some environmental noise perception may linger for a while. The point when such losses become 'deafness' depends greatly on the individual – that is, on when he concedes to the increasing difficulties. Depending on how he uses his hearing, he may experience his hearing loss as a progression: no more listening to radio news, then no longer using the phone, then starting to use television captions instead of loud volume, and so on. For people with progressive deafness, the early adjustment phases we discuss in Chapter 2 are very significant. A person with progressive hearing loss, especially loss that starts in youth, may not identify strongly with 'hearing' people, so that he always feels himself apart from the hearing world. He may develop satisfactory deaf functional skills (i.e., elaborate ways of faking comprehension), but have no discernable prompt to change his self-image from hearing to deaf.

1.3.5 Psychiatric

Psychiatric hearing loss, in our sense of the term, is also found in a medical classification system, among the 'functional' categories.[11] There is really only one kind of genuinely psychiatric deafness, and it is called a Conversion Disorder.[12] The 'conversion,' in this case to being deaf, serves to resolve some unconscious psychological conflict and to keep the conflict out of awareness (for example, to a person abused as a child, becoming deaf would shut out the sounds that could bring back these painful memories). No hearing means no conflicts: this direct link is referred to as a 'primary gain.' Or perhaps the individual enjoys some benefit or avoids some undesirable obligation by acquiring the symptoms, but the link is unconscious: this is referred to as a 'secondary gain.' A patient with conversion deafness is not fabricating the symptoms. She really cannot 'hear,' no matter that in neurological terms, her hearing is intact.

Some people may become 'deaf' for psychological reasons, even though they actually *can* hear, at least a little, and know they can. Some of these people hear perfectly well and are only pretending to be deaf. Others are hard of hearing but have decided quite deliberately that they would rather be counted among the deafened. (We are excluding here people who believe mistakenly that they have been deafened, because they don't fully understand the diagnosis they have been provided or because they have been given poor advice.) An inappropriate desire to portray a more severe hearing loss may be the result of bad experiences among hard-of-hearing people. Or it may stem from the idea of secondary gain – that is, from the belief that deaf people get more latitude, admiration, friends, sympathy, charity, or tax benefits. This latter is referred to as Malingering or Factious Disorder. In Conversion Disorder, the link between the symptoms and the secondary gain is unconscious; in Malingering or Factious Disorder, it is conscious.[13] (Clinically speaking, *malingering* refers to to the production of symptoms that are understandable given the situation; thus, it is understandable to prefer a better support group and better tax benefits. A *factious* disorder is motivated only by the desire to assume the role of a sick person.)

People with a malingering or factious disorder are occasionally caught out. They are rarely remorseful, and sometimes they don't even stop. Fortunately, these cases are rare. Out of the hundreds of self-identified deafened people we have known, we've encountered only one person with a possible conversion disorder, and a handful who showed any signs of a malingering or factious disorder. Without exaggerating the prevalence of this category, we would advise counsellors and support groups that such people might come along.

1.4 Prevalence

As we pointed out earlier, the only available data on hearing loss onset indicate that 75 per cent of adults who are deaf did not become deaf until after the age of nineteen.[14] In the National Deaf Census, the rate of deafened adults was 670 per 100,000 population, or 1 in every 150 people. For Canada, which has a population of 30 million,[15] this translates to 201,000 deafened adults; for the United States, which had a population of 258 million in 1993,[16] this translates to 1,728,600 deafened adults! Yet the Association of Late-Deafened Adults consistently has fewer than 500 paying members, including those residing outside the United States. See Table 1.1 for percentages at different degrees of loss as reported in different references; these proportions can be applied to the population base of the reader's choice.

A major criticism of the body of work on deafened adults, and on 'adventitious' or 'acquired' hearing loss, is that the definitions have been inconsistent. One study found that among those who self-reported a hearing loss, 46 per cent turned out to be false-positives when audiometric follow-up was done, and 17 per cent turned out to be false-negatives.[17] Self-reported hearing loss is apparently an unreliable indicator. Some major studies have included subjects with only moderate hearing losses, drawn from rosters of hearing aid clinics. This 'dilutes' the sample with people who have substantial residual hearing and may be able to cope quite well; it also places those with profound hearing loss in a small minority. Those with the most profound hearing loss (i.e., those who don't have hearing aids, because they would be useless) would not have been included at all. Our point here is that incidence rates are confounded by sampling from populations that do not properly represent the extent of acquired deafness. The only 'encouraging' observation is that these studies have found significant adjustment difficulties even among those with moderate and severe degrees of hearing loss.

The causes of both congenital and adventitious deafness have changed over time. The illnesses of infancy and childhood are now more likely to be prevented, or diagnosed and treated before deafness results. At the same time, genetic screening for the causes of late-onset deafness, such as NF–2, is more readily available, as are public health programs that can reduce the incidence of deafness caused by bacteria and viruses. On the other hand, industrial and environmental noise sources are on the increase; noise-induced hearing loss could be expected to follow. And as modern society grows more hectic, the possibilities for traumatic injury are increasing. A properly administered epidemiology of deafness would end

TABLE 1.1
Prevalence of hearing loss

Segment	Proportion of total population	Source (see bibliography)
Hearing loss	9.74%	Adams & Benson, 1991
Some degree of hearing impairment	10	House, 1999
≥25 dB loss in better ear (South Australia)	16.6	Wilson et al. 1999
≥25 dB loss in better ear (U.K.)	16.1	Davis, 1989 cited in Wilson et al. 1999
Hard of hearing		
Hearing loss 'sufficient to make it difficult or impossible to hear a normal conversation'	4	Levitt & Bakke, 1995
Need help (surgical or amplification) to hear	1	House, 1999
Moderate loss (≥45 dB in better ear, South Australia)	2.8	Wilson et al. 1999
Moderate loss (≥45 dB in better ear, U.K.)	3.9	Davis, 1989 cited in Wilson et al. 1999
Moderate loss (≥45 dB in better ear) age 71+ (S. Aust.)	21.4	Wilson et al. 1999
Moderate loss (≥45 dB in better ear) age 71+ (U.K.)	17.6	Davis, 1989 cited in Wilson et al. 1999
Hard of hearing with aging		
Loss ≥40 dB, hospital continuing care patients	72	Woodcock, 1988
Loss ≥20 dB, nursing home residents	83	Cdn. Hearing Society, 1987
Some degree of hearing loss > age 65	33	House, 1999
Deaf (Normally ≥70 dB for 'severe,' 90 dB for 'profound')		
Severe (≥65 dB loss in better ear)	0.5	Wilson et al. 1999
Deaf prelingual	0.035–0.3	Sneed & Joss, 1999
Deaf all ages, including prelingual	0.873	Sneed & Joss, 1999
'Totally deaf'	0.1	House, 1999
Deafened after age 19	0.68	Schein & Delk, 1974
Age at onset of hearing loss		Unpublished data from participants at ALDAcon 1993
0–10*	14.2%	
11–20*	11.1	
21–30	30.1	
31–40	15.8	
41–50	19.0	
51+	9.5	

*Respondents considered themselves deafened despite prevocational age at onset.

the selection bias inherent in past surveys and eliminate linguistic and technical barriers to measuring the true prevalence of deafness in all its forms.

We are also concerned about neglecting deafened adolescents. 'Hearing loss in adults' has been used as a synonym for late deafness. Both of us were deafened before the age of nineteen and would be classified as 'prevocationally deaf' in the deaf census; yet from the perspective of adjustment, we clearly fit into the 'deafened' rather than the 'born deaf' category.

1.4.1 Prevalence across Classifications

Figure 1.3 illustrates the rates of different causes among deafened people. A 1984 survey of over 100 people conducted by the National Association of Deafened People (NADP) in the U.K. indicated that over 57 per cent were deafened from medical and surgical causes, almost 4 per cent from accidents, and 13.4 per cent from congenital/familial causes. (The remainder were 'unknown'; for these people, the causes are more likely to be hereditary.)[18] In 1994–5, the Association of Late-Deafened Adults (ALDA) conducted its own survey. Among the respondents, 41.5 per cent reported progressive losses, including the apparently hereditary; 40.5 per cent had medical losses; almost 13 per cent had surgical losses; and about 5 per cent became deaf as a result of a traumatic injury.[19]

These figures should be interpreted cautiously. The samples were not drawn from the general population; to be included in these samples, someone had to already be a known deafened person on a mailing list somewhere. In this type of study, people hiding in their closets afraid to go out, and other isolated deafened people, are not going to receive questionnaires. If any type of deafness was more likely to cause people to withdraw from others, the proportions of that type could be underrepresented. The memberships of deafened and other deaf organizations are a tiny fraction of the deafened population, as estimated from the proportions found in the National Deaf Census.

Figure 1.3: Prevalence of hearing loss origin among surveyed members of deafened people's associations

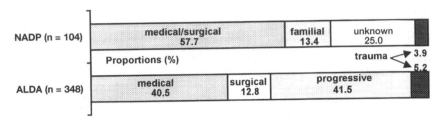

1.5 Judgments of Deafness

Quite apart from the measurements of *hearing*, which is the functional capacity of the auditory perception system we described earlier, we must consider the judgment of *deafness*. Because of the variety of reasons people become deaf, and the rates and ages of onset, there is much confusion about who is actually 'deaf.' A hearing loss can be mild, moderate, severe, or profound. Some people are born deaf or with a hearing loss, while others experience all or part of their hearing loss later. We'll refer to mild or moderate (or monaural – i.e., one-sided) hearing loss as 'hard of hearing' and define that as outside the scope of this book. We will *not* exclude anyone on the basis of age. You do not have to make it into adulthood with intact hearing to be 'late' deafened. However, if you became deaf in early childhood and were educated as a deaf child, then we'll define that as outside the scope of discussion. We *will* include those who grew up hard of hearing and became deaf later, those who lost their hearing early but were educated in the hearing mainstream pretty much untouched by concessions to deafness, and those who experienced all of their hearing loss in the teen years or later.

1.5.1 Various Tests of Deafness

This section discusses the different 'tests' applied to determine whether an individual is *deaf*. We also provide some personal observations as to the relevance and practical application of each 'test.'

All you hear is total silence. This is the strictest auditory criterion. Typically, this standard isn't used clinically or culturally, but it's sometimes what hearing people imagine deafness to be like.

Rare as it is, total silence is a very convincing indicator. If you had neurofibromatosis-related surgery and the surgeon removed your auditory nerves, you're probably not asking questions about whether you are really deaf. Go directly past all this soul searching.

You can't hear the phone. This is a somewhat more flexible standard and was an early definition proposed by ALDA.

The 'telephone test,' once proposed as the litmus test for deafness, is not as clear-cut as it seems. Some deaf people can use a regular telephone in stilted and highly controlled ways, so let's not take 'can't hear the phone' too literally. If you *are* deaf, you can't just pick up a ringing telephone with confidence that you'll understand the person who is calling. But you shouldn't consider yourself disqualified from deafness if you can pluck up the nerve to dial your wife's office (hoping like hell that no one else answers) and carry on a conversation by having her paraphrase every sentence several times, answer yes or no to your questions, or use the spelling trick (see below). Don't feel too guilty about using the phone and still saying you're deaf.

Deafened people seemed to spontaneously invent the spelling trick without discussing it among themselves. If you've never used it, here's how it works. Your wife, let's say, says a word, and (of course) you don't get it. For example, she asks you to pick some (two syllable word) on your way home from work. You ask her to spell out this item, but not the regular way, as in 'pick up the b–a–b–y' (because you could mis-hear that as d–k–t–i and still be confused). The spelling trick involves spelling the mystery word 'pick up the a–*b, a*, a–*b*, a–b–c–d–e–f–g–h–i–j–k–l–m–n–o–p–q–r–s–t–u–v–w–x– *y.*' In some conversations, all the words are mystery words. It gets worse if they have a lot of letters or make use of a lot of letters from the end of the alphabet. With any luck, you might recognize the word from the number of syllables plus the context, plus the first bit of the spelling. That's with luck. It could have been b–r–a–t–w–u–r–s–t instead of b–a–b–y. It doesn't make you not-deaf if you can have an oral conversation this way. It's not like you're going to phone someone to ask for a job and say, 'Sorry, I didn't catch what you said. Could you repeat that by spelling each word from the beginning of the alphabet to each letter in sequence?'

You rely on visual information instead of audible information. This is a more contemporary definition, and is the one favoured by ALDA.

If you 'feel' that you can hear but the sound disappears when you close your eyes, you've probably been lipreading more than you realized. I also have the inverse: if I can see it, I imagine it makes a sound. I can even 'hear' insects crawling. When you're visual, you understand television plots much better when the captions are displayed, and retain the name of a person you've just met when you can read a name tag instead of just an oral introduction. I was visual for twenty years before I figured out I was deaf, though. I recall annoying my Conversational French teacher in Grade 4, demanding that she spell *fenêtre*, an unlipreadably guttural word. Written French was supposed to be of no consequence in her quest to help us acquire the language naturally, but I needed it in writing to make sure I caught the word properly.

K.W.

You don't function in the 'hearing' world. An audiologist's guideline. This rule is usually applied in the inverse to determine who is hard of hearing as opposed to deaf.

When I asked my audiologist if I was deaf, he said there were no audiological thresholds to define deafness. His profession preferred functional definitions. Since I functioned in the hearing way (he observed), I would be called hard of hearing rather than deaf. I was sitting in his little airless booth, holding my breath to try to pluck pure tones and spondee (two-syllable words) out of the headphones, and basically not doing well at all. I could hear a high-decibel 500 Hz tone and that was it for pure tones. We did some sentence tests through the window between our booths and I scored perfect when I was looking at him, sound or no sound. He expressed amazement that I passed for hearing as I did, yet because I didn't know any other way to function, he told me I was hard of hearing. A year later, I had learned enough sign language to take interpreters to business meetings and academic conferences, and I was stunned by how much more I comprehended with a year's sign language study compared to twenty years of lipreading experience.

After years of reflection, the functional definition strikes me as rather circular. A person needs to have the option before you can infer that she has chosen to function in a particular way. I functioned orally because that's all I knew. And in retrospect, for a long time it was only half function, and half fakery.

K.W.

You can't hear beyond certain auditory thresholds. This is a quantitative, audiometric standard, now apparently out of fashion in hearing clinics.

A single hearing-loss number is based on the average hearing threshold at three frequencies: 500 Hz, 1 kHz, and 2 kHz (these three cover the main speech spectrum of 300 to 3000 Hz). For each ear, at these three frequencies, you take the average of the quietest audible decibel level. The ear with the lowest number (smallest hearing loss) is called the Better Ear, and the average decibel hearing loss at those three frequencies is the Better Ear Average (BEA). If your BEA is 90 dB or more you're profoundly deaf, if 70 to 90 dB you're severely deaf, and onward up the chart to moderate or mild. Frankly, this calculation appeals to me more than the functional definition because it gave me permission to yield to the huge burden of a 90 dB loss.

Auditory threshold is not necessarily the best test of deafness for everyone. My ability to pass for hearing right up to 90 dB was enabled by my very slow rate of hearing loss and thus my opportunity to hone my lipreading (and faking) skills over twenty years. Someone who is whacked on the head in a mugging and loses 65 dB overnight may be so disrupted by the difference that oral functioning is out of the question.

K.W.

Always been deaf, went to a deaf school, had deaf parents.
The Deaf Culture's criterion, almost as strict as total silence.

The first question Deaf strangers ask each other is, 'What school did you go to?' Among those who qualify, those from Deaf families are the élite, the 'Deaf of Deaf.' Obviously, the majority of deafened people are not going to pass these traditional Deaf Culture tests, even though some deafened people have been deaf longer than the deaf youngsters who sneer at their pedigree. There are some people whose hereditary late deafness has been dominant in their family tree, and there are some whose adolescent moderate hearing loss got them into a deaf and hard-of-hearing classroom. Most deafened people are at a disadvantage in these 'seniority-based' definitions. This is unfortunate when it comes to role models. Deafened people wake up in the morning just as deaf as those who have been deaf longer. Because of the opportunities they had pre-deafness, they often have attained impressive jobs. When they continue doing those jobs, it proves that deafness alone is not a barrier to doing those jobs. But as long as there is discrimination within the deaf population, nothing is likely to come of the great potential for collaboration with role models.

It seems that this test is applied mainly to the living. Dead deaf people automatically become deaf enough, such as Girl Scouts founder Juliette Gordon Low, the composer Beethoven, the inventor Edison, and so on.

Cannot rely on your natural or aided hearing to effectively comprehend spoken information in environments and situations where people normally can. We consider *deaf* any person who cannot rely on hearing for comprehension in most reasonable environments (i.e., where most people can rely on hearing). Regardless of the measurable amount of residual hearing, if you cannot use it effectively, we shall consider you deaf. Regardless of your lack of skills to function the deaf way, we shall consider you deaf if the sole option of functioning the hearing way is unreliable. We consider *deafened* any person who used to be able to rely on hearing for comprehension but who no longer can. We include those who needed to adjust to deafness from normal hearing, as well as those who used to function with limited, possibly aided, hearing but who no longer find it a reliable means of comprehension. Thus, 'deaf' relates to the capacity for reliable auditory information reception, and 'deafened' refers to a significant change from a former to a current state.

1.5.2 Hearing Impaired

Some past studies have referred to deafened people and acquired hearing loss as an omnibus category, using criteria such as eligibility for hearing aid prescriptions or some moderate or severe decibel level of loss. The result has been that people with substantial 'oral/aural' function have been included in the group. This book is not addressed to people at all levels of acquired hearing loss. We are not addressing those who can hear with difficulty if they have appropriate amplification (hearing aids) or if they escape loud background noise, although they and their counsellors may find this book helpful. Instead, we are focusing on people who cannot make reliable, practical use of any residual hearing they may have.

This is not a book about 'the hearing impaired.' Often, people who are neither deaf nor hard of hearing use the term 'hearing impaired' in a way that brings both audiological populations under the same umbrella. Usually it seems that convenience is the only motivation for combining the two. Unfortunately, this usage ignores the fact that the two groups differ in almost all aspects except the anatomical location of their difference from 'normal.' This is not a matter of political correctness, although it does suggest a more sensitive approach. The 'h.i.' term is imprecise and meaningless. We have no quarrel with 'hearing impairment' as a condition that is possessed by someone; but when we talk of conditions, we prefer to refer to 'deafness' or 'hearing loss,' whichever is appropriate. As we will show in the upcoming chapters, it is the loss, and not merely the impairment or the deafness, that occupies centre stage in the deafened person's experience.

The term 'hearing impaired' is often used by people who don't want to deal with their deafness or hearing loss, and by people who want to dominate those who are deaf or have a hearing loss. People who say they are hearing impaired tend to be afraid to say they are deaf, or they are hard of hearing but don't like that term.

1.6 Impairment, Disability, Handicap, Function

Rehabilitators[20] and the World Health Organization[21] have defined the key concepts of impairment, disability, and handicap in a pertinent and effective way that puts the term impaired in an anatomical context, disability in a task context, and handicap in a social context.[22] In this scheme of things, 'disability' or 'handicap' is an ecological statement about an individual in an environment. Disability may reflect not only the task environment but also the social environment. Thus, an economic need for more workers may cause society's threshold of disability to shift upwards in severity.[23]

A body structure or function (or both) that deviates from generally accepted population standards constitutes an impairment (in some writings, referred to as a 'defect' or an 'abnormal part'). This deviation may be rated in severity from mild to a total absence of function, but it must be detectable or noticeable.

Every person is able to perform a spectrum of activities. People also may experience some activity limitations. Limitations of activities are equivalent to disability. Note that a limitation, or disability, does not mean incapacitation, but rather that a conventional means to accomplish a goal cannot be used. It is possible that an alternative or modified activity can accomplish the same goal. The most significant feature of both classifications is that the impairment of body structure or function is a characteristic of the person but disability resides in the activity. If there is no need to perform the activity, or if there is an alternative, then the impairment is of little consequence. Furthermore, the disability (or limitation of activities) does not in itself constitute a 'handicap.'

A participation restriction or handicap occurs as a result of a combination of factors, including body structure and function, activity restrictions, and physical, social, and attitudinal environments.

A person who is deafened has an impairment. (He may have several impairments, but at minimum he will have some deficiency in the structure and/or function of the hearing apparatus.) He undertakes a spectrum of activities by choice and obligation. If none of those chosen or required activities depends on hearing, then the impairment is more or less inconsequential.

I stood weeping at the ground transport console at Dallas–Fort Worth Airport, utterly confounded by how to make a shuttle van come and get me. The airport courtesy desks were closed for the evening and the ground transport/hotel console was the usual 'lift receiver and press button corresponding to your hotel' model. Here I was, arriving in town to present a keynote address at a conference, the supreme example of 'the achiever,' and I couldn't even get from the airport to the hotel because of someone's assumptions about what capabilities people were supposed to have.

K.W.

Thus, a deafened person whose job requires him to respond by e-mail to customer service requests received through a website is not limited by the impairment at work.

If his activities are restricted, or if they have been modified so that he can perform them – but he does perform them – then he has a disability but no handicap. For instance, he may use TTY/relay to communicate with hearing people whom he cannot talk to on a voice telephone. Disability, then, reflects not only the impairment but also the need to use a modified means of access, due to the non-use of universal design.

If no tools can be made, and if no modifications of existing tools are possible, that will enable a person to perform required activities, and if that person is limited in her participation in society and in normal life, then she has a handicap. In other words, a handicap reflects the lack of availability of tools to enable access. There are so many rehabilitation and access aids available for deaf people that it would be unusual to consider a deaf person handicapped unless she had additional impairments or had goals that could only be achieved with hearing centred activities. We believe that the key to ensuring participation, and to preventing and reducing restrictions, lies in task design and reasonable accommodation.

No one is handicapped merely by virtue of his own characteristics. There are no 'disabled people' – however, due to design practices and social conventions, there are some people who encounter restrictions more often than others.[24] Society creates restrictions, or handicaps, when it fails to remove barriers or to provide facilitation. Even a person with fully 'normal' body function and structure can best be described using a term coined by the disability access movement: 'temporarily able bodied.' A person who enjoys unrestricted participation cannot rely on remaining that way.

Chapter 2

Adjustment to Deafness

As they appear both in biographies and in academic literature reviews, descriptions of acquired deafness are a virtual thesaurus for the word 'catastrophe': thunderbolt, shattering, calamitous, disastrous, traumatic, devastating. The focus is usually on the utter enormity of the impediment, if not its absolute insurmountability. These descriptions are designed to convince the reader that the condition, though invisible, is not insignificant. But there is a paradox here: the descriptions are based on reports of survivors, so evidently the catastrophe is surmountable after all. Rather than describing how people have survived ten or twenty years beyond, these resources focus on the period of trauma and loss, and serve mainly to provide the dimensions of the devastation. It is more valuable to understand the adjustment process than to merely sympathize with the catastrophe. This chapter discusses the lengthy, complicated process of adjustment from a variety of perspectives.

2.1 Acquired Deafness, Acquired Stigma

An individual who is disqualified from full social acceptance on the basis of some less desirable attribute has been stigmatized.[1] It might sound self-pitying to appropriate the status of 'stigmatized,' but our personal experience and observation has convinced us that Erving Goffman's description of stigma does much to explain the impact that deafness has. If we are to appreciate the responses that deafened adults have to becoming deaf, it is important that we understand the phenomenon of stigma, and that is why this chapter and the next owe a great deal to Goffman's work. A stigma incorporates the attribute itself and the associated undesirable attributes. The way the stigma term is used metaphorically illustrates the implications. Everyone has heard the word *deaf* used in these contexts: 'Are you deaf or something?' 'These reasonable suggestions fell on deaf ears.' In the stigma sense, deafness is interpreted as incorporating stupidity and unreasonable stubbornness.

The aversion toward hearing aids as a symbol of hearing loss stigma is so well known that invisibility is used as a marketing angle for entirely-in-the-canal aids. British member of Parliament Jack Ashley, deafened within his first two years in office, was determined not to use sign interpreting, even though he recognized that it could give him complete access, 'so there would be no contrast with other people.'[2]

Society has its views on how a stigmatized person should make 'a good adjustment.' It encourages and rewards those who adapt best, meaning those who appear to differ least from 'normal,' meaning (often) those who do not think of themselves as disabled and do not interact much with others who have a disability. The specimens of good adjustment, the 'folk heroes of disease,'[3] are those who conceal their disability so well that no one becomes conscious of it until after they have attained their success – those few who *overcome* their disability (and thereby create the perception that any disabled person who does not adjust just doesn't have the same strength of character).

Stigmatized people are typically advised to view 'normals' as well-meaning, and to take responsibility for breaking the ice and making other people comfortable with their condition, and to act appreciative of others' efforts to help them. The stigmatized person is also expected to be sensitive to the limits of society's tolerance and not to push too far; and to avoid situations that would impose an excessive burden, or make others uncomfortable, or force them to confront the truth about the limits to their tact and tolerance. Of course, all of this directly contradicts society's outward insistence that the condition is no cause for sadness or shame or concealment, but merely an inconvenience to be borne cheerfully.

Those who meet these expectations are perceived as having 'strong character.' However, from the point of view of stress, maintaining a 'positive attitude' is not the same as 'adapting well.' It can be unhealthy to externally and internally portray this image of good adjustment. When we suppress negative emotions, we decrease our ability to experience either positive or negative emotions. Expressing negative emotions (anger and so on) along with realistic optimism actually improves survival in life-threatening situations such as cancer.[4]

For some people, the cause of stigma becomes the primary explanation for all sorts of failings and disappointments. Every rejection or hardship seems to be brought on by deafness. Alternatively, deafness can be seen by some as a blessing in disguise and an exercise in character-building to prepare the individual for some higher calling. People who are not disabled may regard people with disabilities as courageous and ingenious, and reflect this in their patterns of interaction. Whether this is simply an expression of admiration or feigned sensitivity, it is often perceived as negative and patronizing by the other party.[5]

> Perhaps I am hypersensitive to discrimination. When I have bad service from a company, I automatically think they don't want deaf customers. I have escalated the confrontation, provoking the business, refusing to talk to them through the telephone relay service and insisting they should have a TTY. It probably isn't fair and it may not be effective, but it has met my immediate emotional needs.
>
> M.A.

People who have or acquire a stigma are aware that others don't fully accept them. Indeed, they may themselves share the dislike for the attribute. Deaf and hard-of-hearing people perceive that others stigmatize them because the others seem impatient, they whisper, they patronize, they seem not to understand about hearing loss, they express how difficult it is to communicate. Feelings of being stigmatized can lead to self-hate: hate for the group to which the stigma has consigned them.

Anticipating the reactions of others can lead to fear and distress and to anxious efforts to prevent those reactions. Goffman explained how those with an undesirable quality often strive to correct the condition, and how they are prone to being victimized.[6] Because they desire so much to escape the stigma, these people tend to embrace any potential remedy. Potential remedies include those not yet on the market; potential may be only alleged. Those who are victimized by the unscrupulous or who make bad choices remain stigmatized. Not only do these aids not correct the condition, but people who try them may feel that their position has worsened if they perceive that it reveals them as gullible. And even if the remedy works, those who take it may succeed only in transferring themselves into a differently stigmatized group: the formerly afflicted – the bionically assisted, for example.[7]

Others respond to their stigma with indirect efforts, by attempting to master what is supposed to be impossible for them. Deafened people may throw themselves passionately into musical or other auditory pursuits in an attempt to show that they are not deaf, or that deafness is not a barrier. Deafened musicians are a staple human interest story on the evening news. Zola, a 'successful' adapter to his disability, pointed out the paradox: that in order to be recognized as having successfully adapted, one must divest oneself of any identification with the condition, and deny the uncomfortable features of that life, because 'to not do so would make our success impossible!'[8] (Even so, he wondered whether he had achieved this only because of his income and position, which made it possible for him to 'command' the resources he needed, and whether those without access to this level of power simply gave up, avoided those encounters, and became isolated.)

Disclosing my deafness has been in some ways good for me because I don't feel that I am always responsible for meeting everyone else 99 per cent of the way. I beat myself up less and am not quite so tired at the end of the day. On the other hand, it has significantly reduced the opportunities available to me. There is no doubt that professional opportunities have become fewer as a result of the perception people have that my deafness would be unworkable. There is no question that various opportunities created for my 'unique' talents have had more than an overtone of 'sheltered workshop' to them. Now, instead of the stress of passing, I have the stress of being diminished. I had it better when I passed, but I don't know for sure that I would have been able to continue passing. It's too late for second-guessing.

K.W.

2.2 Complication with Other Problems

Contrary to the proposition that deafened people should not be excessively bitter because 'everyone has their problems,' deafened people are not given a free pass out of life's other difficulties. Deafened people break legs, suffer heart attacks, and go into labour the same as normal-hearing people do, except that they have to get through these challenges with impeded communication with caregivers. We could argue that deafened people run a higher risk for other adversities in those situations where health promotion and public health and emergency warning information doesn't get through due to deafness.

The same traumatic injury that caused the deafness may cause other permanent damage. Or the virus that caused the hearing loss may cause chronic fatigue or recurring viral episodes. Clearly, the deafness that appears with advanced age is only one of the many age-related medical problems that people may encounter.

There are many medical syndromes for which deafness is just one of several symptoms. Depending on the specific disorder, deafness may be accompanied by visual disturbances or by blindness, balance disorders, kidney disease, or spinal tumours. When you consider that visual channels are the main means of adapting to deafness, it's clear that people who become deaf *and* blind face huge practical challenges. These are beyond the scope of this book, although the emotional processes may be similar. In keeping with the aims of this book, we will not review the list of such syndromes (even if we could do it justice). Our aim is to emphasize that family, friends, and professionals should not imply that a deafened person should 'lighten up, because everyone has their troubles.' Deafness is not a get-out-of-jail-free card for other health problems. If anything, a greater prevalence of other problems should be presumed.

2.2.1 *Psychological*

Deafened people are also at risk to mental health problems. A variety of psychological studies and reviews[9] have suggested that people with hearing loss can develop paranoia, depression, withdrawal, irritability, fatigue, nervousness, and feelings of isolation. The family's well-meaning efforts to cheer them up may cause extra irritation, possibly precipitating emotional collapse. One sees fear of failure and ridicule, of being slighted and avoided, of people and new situations, of sudden noises or imagined sounds. One encounters feelings of worthlessness, shame, rage, despondency, and suspicion, and perhaps even suicidal feelings. Of course, everyone has some of these feelings to some degree at some point. In one study, people with hearing losses over 70 dB had significantly higher scores for anxiety and depression, not just compared to people who enjoyed normal hearing, but compared to people who had milder hearing losses![10]

It is only logical that the risk of depression increases when there is social isolation or a perceived lack of social support. Both are common during a person's transition from hearing to not hearing. Cutting off communication and the channel of information seems to be enough to cause depression, although of course, depression is also associated with other stigmas.[11] A person can easily become suspicious, depressed, hostile, anxious, and bewildered in the absence of positive feedback, when self-imposed isolation replaces socializing. Anxiety and feelings of insecurity and inferiority arise from fear of others' disrespect. The individual may have heightened awareness of the stigma while believing that others feel no self-consciousness. Quite aside from the loss of communication and access to warning signals that ensure personal security, deafness is a deprivation of the primitive background – those environmental sounds that affirm one is alive.[12]

Anxiety and depression increase the risk that an individual will 'self-medicate' – that is, try to alleviate these through the use of alcohol or drugs – and perhaps engage in other dysfunctional behaviours such as overeating. There is no reason to believe that deafened people are immune to this risk. In one study, rates of alcoholism and self-reported heavy drinking were higher among older, employed people with hearing impairments than among those with normal hearing.[13] It seems logical to assume that the effect would be most pronounced among those experiencing a severe or profound loss of hearing, especially if this is coupled with a disruption of employment. (This study consolidated new, old, mild, and severe hearing impairments into one category, 'hearing impaired'; while people without employment were excluded.)

Moreover, a deafened person who already had alcoholism or addiction prior to becoming deaf now has one more obstacle to overcome before recovering from the substance abuse. Few '12-step programs' (e.g., Alcoholics Anonymous)[14] exist for deaf people, and almost all of these are oriented to the sign-language users in the Deaf culture. Thus, the deafened person is bounced from the mainstream because he can't hear and is then bounced from the margins because he can't sign, and falls through the cracks. This compounds the isolation that led to the anxiety or depression in the first place.

> Even though I could sign, my deaf 12-step group could not comprehend me when I tried to talk about my feelings of isolation and loss related to deafness. To them, being deaf was the very thing that created and defined and cemented their social circles. For me, it was what cut me off. We had a mutually awkward relationship and eventually I withdrew.
>
> M.A.

These extreme and undesirable psychological responses are quite normal and logical when one considers the experience of deafened adults. It is hard to criticize paranoia when people really are talking about you behind your back, or fear of ridicule when your dignity is repeatedly undermined by people making 'good natured' jokes, and intentionally covering their mouths and sharing stories where your misunderstanding of something was funny. An *absence* of vulnerability or any sense of dignity might be more unusual. To avoid adverse consequences from these feelings, the deafened person must work through them and adapt to the new reality. Perhaps deafened people can only achieve a 'normal' psychological state with respect to deafened norms.

2.3 What Is Normal for Deafened Adults?

Past reports on late deafness[15] have described various common experiences, phenomena, and reactions but do not help us interpret how the adjustment is progressing. In one model, the phase that follows the prescription of a hearing aid is one 'open-ended' stage.[16] Its beginning is marked by abandonment of the struggle for control. Otherwise, there are no specific behavioural or identity benchmarks.[17] Without a more structured guide, the counsellor may be unable to gauge whether an individual is progressing, regressing, overreacting, or becoming mired in difficulties. Our aim is to describe how adjustment evolves as the client's identity changes from hearing to deafened. We have created a holistic model incorporating various models. To this, we have added metaphors to describe various stable states, into which the client may settle and stop evolving.

2.3.1 Background on the Bereavement Model for Hearing Loss

Many social workers and people working with deafened adults are familiar with applying the stages of grief or bereavement to the process. Perhaps the best-known model of grief, and one that is often applied to deafness,[18] is that of Kübler-Ross,[19] who wrote of how people prepare themselves for death in stages. The most commonly used version of the stages goes as follows: denial, anger, bargaining, depression, and acceptance. Kübler-Ross later came to assert that this stages model could apply to any form of loss, from spouse to job to contact lenses.[20] Amid emerging criticism of Kübler-Ross's methods,[21] we prefer Parkes's model dealing with the loss of a loved one.[22] Deafness, like widowhood, imposes a loss on a life that must continue. There is no inevitable, foreseeable point of reckoning when grieving – and life – ends; rather the loss involves an indefinite 'life sentence.' The most noteworthy finding of Parkes's research was that favourable adjustment to widowhood depends on social support. Hearing loss interferes with such support: the very thing a person needs in order to deal with bereavement – communication – is precisely what has been lost. This model would predict that most people confronted with hearing loss will have difficulty adapting successfully. The fact that many adaptations do succeed seems contrary to that model as interpreted directly.

Some deafened people seem to have experienced bereavement and recall feelings of denial, anger, and so on. Others report that they did not, and that they experienced more of an identity struggle. This variation may relate to how rapidly deafness occurred, and other individual differences. Those who have a sudden loss and/or are in a stage of life where stability is expected may be disposed to a traumatic response and bereavement; those who are in a flexible stage of life, and those who experience a very gradual progressive hearing loss, may relate to their deafness as an identity shift.

> In my deafened support group, everyone else was an over-nighter, coping with new ways of functioning, mourning absent music. They were sure they were deaf, and didn't know how to cope. I knew how to function, but wasn't sure I was deaf.
>
> K.W.

Identity change is illustrated exceptionally well by the 'coming out' process of gay/lesbian people. In a number of ways, the self- and public acknowledgment of homosexuality is similar to the process of accepting one's deafness. Both are processes of dis-identification that involve breaking away from a prescribed behaviour or role in society and accepting an identity that entails a stigma. Coming out happens in a series of stages, at the end of which a gay/lesbian person assumes a homosexual identity both privately and publicly.[23] In accepting one's deafness, the formerly hearing identity is replaced with a deaf identity.

While there are differences in the language used, identity change and bereavement have several parallels, and we have thus integrated them into a unified model, which we call 'the model of deafened adjustment.'

2.3.2 Progression through the Stages

A difficulty with multistage models is the presumption that stages represent a norm: a 'right' way to adjust and a 'destination' that all 'properly adjusted' people will attain. In fact, there are many differences, and many reasons for them. People have different rates of hearing loss, so that except in cases of sudden deafness, the point of onset is often highly subjective. Many factors affect when a deafened person will recognize her hearing loss and begin the adjustment process. One person will remain for a long time at a particular stage; another will transit rapidly through that same stage but linger in the next. When it comes to adversity, whatever the kind, people have different degrees of vulnerability and resilience.

Progression may depend on the degree to which deafness threatens individual needs.[24] One person may be *traumatized* by a certain degree of hearing loss if it infringes on a central emotional need, such as for safety, intimacy, or power; another person with an objectively greater hearing loss may be merely *stressed* if none of his central emotional needs is seriously threatened. Those with a lesser degree of trauma will progress more readily from stage to stage. These individual differences have been called 'strength of character ... mental, spiritual, and economic resources to triumph over adversity ...'[25]

Antonovsky's Sense of Coherence concept[26] associates successful coping with three components: comprehensibility, manageability, and meaningfulness. *Meaningfulness* is the sense that taking on challenges is worthwhile. If a person lacks a sense of meaningfulness, it will be hard for the other components to compensate, for the motivation to cope will be low. The second most important component is *comprehensibility.* Being able to predict or at least explain circumstances can make adversity more coherent. Third, *manageability* refers to a person's sense of having the resources at her disposal to deal with circumstances. Meaningfulness does not require that the activity be gratifying – merely that it be valued. Comprehensibility doesn't require that the underlying order be fair – merely that it be explicable. Manageability does not mean that the person needs to be able to handle circumstances unaided – merely that the required aid be there, from medical specialists, one's religion, one's significant other, and so on.

Antonovsky believed that sadly, those with a weak sense of coherence are rarely able to increase their sense of coherence through life. Those with a strong sense of coherence perceive themselves as empowered to tackle adversity, feeling as they do that things always worked out in the past; the positive, coherent results of their interventions confirm this belief. A weak sense of coherence leads to a passive response, which produces results that serve to confirm that adversity is arbitrary and that the situation is hopeless. Antonovsky did recognize that the sense of coherence fluctuated about the individual's mean. To maximize the individual's sense of coherence, planned interventions should at the very least ensure that they do not trigger a downward deviation. Furthermore, they should perhaps aim to elicit an elevated sense of coherence, even if the effect is transient. For instance, validating a person's concerns and dissatisfactions can increase his sense of coherence temporarily, by extending a sense of participation (meaningfulness) and commonality (comprehensibility).

Different life circumstances affect the transit time for various stages, by affecting the costs and benefits of staying still or moving on. The sense that a transition is happening 'on time' can alleviate the stress normally associated with change. This openness to change at certain times may reduce the stress of unwanted transitions, such as deafness, that happen to be occurring simultaneously. In one study, people deafened in the first two decades of life credited deafness with increasing their patience; they also expressed more 'gusto' for life – something that seemed to elude those deafened later.[27]

It is inappropriate to apply one model rigidly to everyone; that being said, the advantage of a 'stages' model is that it provides the counsellor with a framework for making suggestions when adjustment seems to be faltering. While our acquaintance with hundreds of deafened people, and personal experience, suggests a general sequence of steps, the later stages are not 'higher' steps on a staircase of improved adjustment. Anyone may find complete satisfaction at any level. Cass used the term 'identity foreclosure' to refer to an individual's choice not to develop any further.[28] There are many practical and functional adjustments that do not require experiencing each of the stages we describe. The deafened person should not feel pressured to behave like someone at a 'more advanced' stage. Such pressure interferes with true adjustment. Remaining at a given stage rather than moving on to a new one is only a problem if it creates perceived problems: we all know we sometimes get 'in a rut' or repeat 'patterns' of mistakes and dissatisfactions. When stagnation does become dysfunctional, this model can show the way forward. A counsellor can use the model, and insight into current and forward stages, to devise stimuli to encourage the client to progress. (Example exercises are provided in Chapter 4, 'Professional Help.')

Steady, one-way progression is not guaranteed: there is nothing that says every deafened person starts 'here' and comes out the other side as a well-adjusted deafened person. A similar process, that of 'coming out,' is not a steady progression through all the stages for every gay man and lesbian, and deafened people are no less diverse. Most people who come out as gay or lesbian will drift back and forth between stages or even return to the beginning of the process after progressing to later stages.[29] This doesn't represent a loss of advances; rather it is a pattern of 'sampling' a more advanced stage and then returning to unfinished business at the earlier stage. This may indicate that the client would respond to the counsellor's help to resolve that unfinished business. Some people will seem to exhibit 'mixed stages' behaviour; in these cases, we suggest that the counsellor try to discern which behaviour is dominant. Apparently regressive behaviours may just be old habits that are hard to break, not a loss of adjustment achievements that have been made.

Smooth progression may also be disrupted by further deterioration in hearing. Many progressive losses take decades. As hearing gradually deteriorates, the individual loses, one at a time, the ability to perform various auditory-based tasks – first the ability to understand song lyrics, then public address announcements, and so on. The residual hearing that helped the deafened person perceive speech cadences and that aided lip-reading disappears, so that it becomes difficult to carry out face-to-face transactions. The perceived misfortune at each stage depends on how important the particular function was in the individual's life circumstances at the time. A person who feels that she is adjusting to deafness may be disarmed by a further

TABLE 2.1
Model of Deafened Adjustment

Stage	Key thoughts	Metaphor
Identity confusion	What is going on?	Not yet ready
Identity comparison	Am I deaf?	Invalid
Identity concession	I am deaf, technically.	Refugee
Identity recognition	I am deaf.	
Deaf activism	I am deaf, dammit!	Religious convert
Depression	I can't change the world.	
Identity synthesis	Acceptance	Immigrant

setback, which in turn may cause her to repeat earlier stages of the adjustment process.

This progression from stage to stage represents the process of adjustment. In addition, we use metaphors in our model to characterize the behaviour of different deafened people who have stabiliized at one of the stages. Specifically, we refer to 'invalids,' 'immigrants,' 'religious converts,' and 'refugees.'

The Model of Deafened Adjustment is summarized in Table 2.1, which shows the sequence of stages, representative thoughts at each stage, and the metaphor for the individual who stabilizes at each stage. In the following section, we describe each of these stages.

2.4 Model of Deafened Adjustment

2.4.1 Identity Confusion:'What Is Going On?'

The onset of deafness can be sudden or progressive. Sudden deafness is when the hearing loss happens overnight (e.g., through injury) or in a very short time (e.g., through illness). With progressive deafness, one's hearing diminishes over months, years, or even (commonly) decades. The *type* of confusion therefore depends on how quickly one becomes deaf.

If the hearing loss occurs spontaneously without any other symptoms – especially if there is still some sound perception – the initial confusion may simply be over the diagnosis. Is this silence, or is it muffled sound due to wax? Or is it a cold? Or is it a repairable injury to the ear? Is it just a hearing loss of normal aging, one that will progress slowly?

With rapid-onset deafness, confusion may arise from the secondary role hearing loss often plays in the overall medical situation. Often, much more attention is devoted to the injuries or illness that occurred with (or caused) the hearing loss. Rather than labelling it 'deafness,' professionals may call it a 'hearing loss,' which sounds milder and implies that the loss may be temporary. People may perceive the hearing difficulties as side effects along the road to recovery from the injury or illness. In cases of sudden deafness, this stage may almost be a trauma or shock event that temporarily paralyses the individual's reaction.

When the hearing loss is progressive, there is no discernable difference from one day to the next, and comparisons from one year to the next are rarely accurate. It is easier to account for functional difficulties by remarking on the situation: 'Nobody can hear with that noise in the background.' 'Nobody can understand public address systems.' The deafened person has no idea what others do hear, and is not alarmed. Since what people say resembles what they hear, effects on pronunciation may be presumed by others to be an accent or, more simply, laziness. Neglect of social cues may be attributed to unfriendliness or snobbishness. Since the family doesn't want to deal with 'deafness' any more than the individual does, often there is no pressure on the individual to clarify the identity confusion. A progressive loss develops its own inertia: Why change something that doesn't really seem all that different?

Why can't I understand public address system announcements? Why are people saying I pronounce words wrong? Why did everyone know about that party but me?

Goffman suggested that the pain of acquiring a disabling condition is not so much from confusion about the new identity;
rather, it arises because the person knows all too well what she
has become.[30] When acquiring a stigma, she will recall all her
own past negative attitudes about it.

With progressive loss, I was able to learn to sign before I lost
my last residual hearing. Transitionally, I was having a comfortable time. I was having problems dealing with *other* people's
issues, but what I couldn't hear was the least of my problems. I
was taken aback, however, when I returned to a major league
ballpark after a three-year hiatus and found that I could no
longer hear the robust bass tones of the national anthems or
the rumble of the crowd. If I'd closed my eyes I could have
been in a meadow. I hadn't imagined it would ever be that
silent, nor had I ever credited how much difference that last little bit of low-frequency sound had been making.

K.W.

The corresponding stage in the bereavement model is *denial*.
For some people, confusion or denial may be a rational
approach to coping: Antonovsky[31] suggested that those with a
strong sense of coherence may interpret stressors as nonprob-
lematic, because in the past things have by and large worked out
well. This is consistent with Zola's[32] observation that those who
deny affiliation with the 'handicapped' group tend to be the
ones perceived as having 'overcome' their condition. It has been
argued that denial plays a positive role, in that it prevents the
individual from prematurely abandoning rewarding activities
that can be continued or modified. This permits him to continue
acquiring other talents that can be of later benefit. Holly Elliott
told of continuing to conduct a half-heard singing choir and
being able to use those conducting skills later to conduct sign
language choirs.[33]

> I was in so much denial that I continued to audition for singing and guitar playing jobs, and enrolled in college to study music. The constant rejection and failure eventually forced me to confront my hearing loss. Unfortunately, I dropped out of college for many years instead of switching to another field. The only 'lasting' asset of my denial stage is a willingness to charge in and embarrass myself. Nothing could be that bad! Even so, I am sensitive to rejection.
>
> M.A.

On the other hand, denial eventually has a price, whether it is fatigue, or accumulated frustration, or the problems related to having publicly committed to never giving in *before* the fullest extent of the hearing loss sets in. Those with progressive losses who adopt the 'deaf' label while still hard of hearing are in some danger of mistakenly believing that the challenge of deafness is exaggerated. We don't really have a metaphor for people becoming stuck at this stage. We just call them 'not yet ready,' in the belief that most will not remain there permanently.

2.4.2 Identity Comparison: 'Am I Deaf?'

Deafened people begin to recognize that other deaf people exist, but they don't identify with those who were born deaf or grew up deaf. At this stage, a deafened person cannot relate to people of Deaf Culture. Although the two types of deafness share common barriers to accessibility in our hearing-centred society, the gap in cultural experiences between late deafness and Deaf Culture is huge. A deaf person is socialized in her family's hearing culture, but a prelingually deaf person acquires culture through residential schools for the deaf,[34] and the differences in language, norms, and values can be as great as those between Afghanistan and Brazil. Should a deafened person, whose signing skills are poor, meet two signing deaf people, the experience is not one that fosters a bonding with them. Instead, it creates deeper feelings of isolation. Elliott wrote that hearing people thought she was hearing because her speech was good and deaf people thought she was hearing because her signs were bad. As a result, she felt caught between incomprehensible speech and incomprehensible signs.[35]

> Many deafened people are deeply pained by the high wall that exists between them and born-deaf culture. Most deafened people find it frustrating to be unable to communicate with the people who are most like them audiometrically. Making the effort to learn how to hurdle this communication barrier and then experiencing rejection is a doubly hurtful experience.

The inability to cope through hearing readily leads to pain and anger. So does having one's identity compared unfavourably with people of the Deaf Culture. 'Why me?' questions are typical of the *anger* phase of the grieving model. Deafened people become angry with themselves and others. For example, a deafened mother in this stage may berate herself for bad mothering after failing to hear her child in distress. She may be angry with family and friends who express frustration at hearing her endless complaints about deafness, or who do not conceal that she is inconveniencing them. Whether or not they express these thoughts, deafened people in this stage form an angry response: 'You can't blame me – it's not my fault this disorder happened to me. If it's inconvenient for you for an hour or a week, how do you think I feel day in and day out?"

> In response to several consecutive audiograms showing a progressive decline, I simply stopped going to the specialist. 'Why bother?' was my thinking. This was a sort of passive-aggressive anger at myself.
>
> K.W.

A client in this stage may visit a social worker, not for help in adjusting to deafness and accepting it, but rather to fix a problem related to unfair work barriers. 'Surely it can't be right that I could lose my job as a switchboard operator, just because I can no longer hear. It isn't fair – I didn't choose this. How can they pick on me? Can I sue them to make them change the job for me?' The immediate problem of income maintenance is an important one for the social worker to address, but this is merely the presenting problem. After the social worker has provided assistance related to it, the client's underlying problems are still there: the only problem that has been fixed is the one the deafened person can bring herself to see and talk about. It is not likely to be the only problem she has, and the social worker needs to use the contact to explore the other impacts that deafness is having. As with many people, her identity may come from her career, and if she is forced out of that, her identity and role are at risk in the other parts of her life.

We use the metaphor 'invalid' when referring to the sickness role adopted here. Deafened people in this stage consider their condition to be a disease or disorder, which leaves room for a remedy. People who need to believe there is an overall fairness in the universe may search for meaning in their predicament – first in medical terms and, failing that, in spiritual terms.

> The same people who don't exercise, and who continue to smoke and eat fatty foods 'because the guidelines are based on inconclusive research,' will beat the doctor's door down when they read in the daily paper that some biologist made a reptile's auditory nerves grow back ... even if it made the reptile's legs fall off and lifespan 25 per cent shorter.

People may remain in the 'invalid' stage for long periods as they search for explanations for their deafness, and for insights into the physiology and anatomy of deafness, and as they seek medical remedies such as surgery and nerve cell regeneration. They bombard Internet discussion groups with questions about

medical treatments and speculation over future cures. They ridicule deafened people for 'giving in' to their deafness and for
joining a low-achieving cohort – which is how they view the
stigmatized deaf population.

> I used to refer to myself as a hearing person trapped in the
> body of a deaf man.
>
> M.A.

As their distaste for deafness persists, and as it begins to sink
in that they truly *have* lost their hearing, deafened people give
various reasons why it is so urgent for their hearing to be
restored: 'I can't expect my friends and family to learn to sign.'
'Interpreters [or real-time reporters] are too expensive for every
deaf person everywhere.' 'I have to work in the hearing world
and it will never adapt to deafness.' In these responses to deafness, one can detect an underlying rejection of the self. In their
view, these reasons are based not on self-rejection but rather on
pragmatism. As the evidence mounts that they are deaf, they
may grasp for identity comparisons with hard-of-hearing people, who share the values of maintaining membership in the
hearing world. Those who settle into the invalid stage are very
likely to seek professional services rather than self-help. Medical,
technological, and legal remedies have strong appeal to them.

> I had a friend who spoke very rapidly and in an elegantly
> accented voice. We carried on an intercontinental correspon-
> dence for ten years, and then she moved back nearby again.
> We met again once. We had got along well during her years
> away, on paper, but when we met again in person, I hadn't a
> clue what she was saying. I never contacted her again.
>
> K.W.

People with a resilient personality, and who receive the

unequivocal professional judgment that their deafness is un-
treatable and irreversible, will progress more rapidly beyond
the identity comparison stage. Also smoothing the process
would be flexibility in personal circumstances (e.g., young and
single), the opportunity to meet other healthy and successful
deaf and particularly deafened people (i.e., so that favourable
comparisons can be made), and the availability of appropriate
rehabilitation and accessibility resources.

A personal experience may push the individual beyond the
identity comparison stage. For example, some people report having been mortified to realize that they replied, 'That's nice,' when
someone told them of the death of a beloved pet. In this example,
lipreading and other oral tools failed, as did the previously reliable coping technique of faking comprehension. Incidents like
this often serve as stimuli for re-evaluating the identity.

When I was first really dealing with hearing loss, I was asking
my audiologist, my sign language teacher, my deaf friends,
and my family, 'Am I deaf?' I was searching for permission,
because it was such a mysterious thing. I had never been deaf,
so I wasn't sure I could recognize it.

For many years during my progressive hearing loss, I
thought deafness was beneath me. Who would I sign with? I
didn't know any of those people. Look at how I was achieving!
Not like *them*. How did I know about *them*? From seeing ped-
dlers. Luckily, I met deaf people who were professionals, like
me. I learned that *fingerspelling* and *selling fingerspelling
cards* were not cause and effect.

It wasn't until I met people with similar progressive hearing
losses that I really felt 'normal': not only our present feelings
but also our memories were identical.

K.W.

2.4.3 Identity Concession: 'I Am Deaf, Technically'

Recognizing that your hearing loss is incontestable does not mean that your concession to deafness is absolute. Conceding that you are deaf 'technically' reflects some uncertainty. Deaf people often reinforce deafened people's impressions that they are not really deaf, by referring to them as 'hard of hearing' or 'a little hard of hearing.' (In Deaf Culture, where the norms are the inverse of the hearing world, 'a little hard of hearing' means 'mainly deaf but with a little hearing.')

A deafened person begins to recognize that she needs to take positive steps to minimize access barriers. She purchases special devices such as TTYs, television closed caption decoders, and flashing alarm systems. This stage can be interpreted as 'bargaining' in the bereavement model: 'If I acquire these devices and practise these behaviours, this discomfort I am feeling may go away.' She may become more selective about social activities, dropping friends who cannot be lipread or who won't be patient. This may be less from annoyance than from a sense of not wanting to 'impose,' reflecting the internalization of stigma.

We use the metaphor 'refugee' for those who remain in this stage. The person has moved to a 'place' with a different character. The relocation may not have been desired or voluntary, but the deafened person has acknowledged that it is better than the possible alternatives. For these people, deafness is similar to being on a trip and losing your passport, being unable to go 'home.'

People who are stuck in the 'refugee' mode may become habitués of support groups. For some, there may be a correspondence between the rewards of the role and their personal values. Those who enjoy being admired for their 'valiant struggle' are likely to remain in this stage longer than others. Their candid sharing of their struggles may be an inspiration to those just entering the identity concession stage; at the same time, however, they may annoy those who have moved on to more advanced stages. Also refugees are those people one finds in deafened clubs who shun support groups but are always ready to advise others on devices and techniques. With their clear-cut answers and universal solutions, these people exhibit what Antonovsky[36] called a *rigid* sense of coherence (as opposed to a strong one). They insist that they have accepted their deafness, yet their acceptance seems to be conditional on their maintaining the precise formula they espouse – perhaps cochlear implants or guide dogs.

Just as the literal refugee aspires to return to his homeland, someday, when the world is a better place, the deafened 'refugee' keeps a deafened ear to the ground for news of treatments that might make this possible.

2.4.4 Identity Recognition: 'I Am Deaf'

The deafened person's progress to Identity Recognition[37] might come about through a gradual loss of patience with the struggle to communicate among hearing people, or through frustration with deaf people continually referring to him as 'hard of hearing' when he feels that hard-of-hearing people cope a lot easier in the hearing world.

In the identity recognition stage, the person internalizes the identity of being deaf, and reorients his core identity so that he is no longer a hearing person who cannot hear, but rather a person who is fundamentally deaf. The deafened person may enrol in sign language courses and, most notably, begin to call himself deaf instead of 'a little hard of hearing' or 'hearing impaired.' He still identifies more with hearing people than with other deaf people, and still thinks often of 'life in the old country'; even so, the dawning of a deaf life has begun.

I stopped hesitating before calling myself deaf, stopped asking permission, and just started doing it. I couldn't tolerate the uncertainty any more, of wondering if I was deaf. If anyone had problems with it, I figured they would say so.

K.W.

The deafened person in the identity concession stage may begin to socialize with deaf people, but the relationship may be one of symbiosis and coexistence more than assimilation. Though a cultural outsider, the deafened person may be accepted in the deaf community because he is 'useful' – for making phone calls, speaking to waiters, explaining government forms, and so on. In return, the deaf club provides social acceptance and the opportunity to improve sign language.

> Despite my increasing fluency in pretty good ASL, I remained an outsider until the deaf club softball team needed a second baseman.
>
> M.A.

Identity recognition is unlikely to be a stable state – that is, most people do not remain in it, but rather bounce back to the refugee state or proceed onward. Whether a person goes forward or back is a matter of individual differences involving resilience, values, opportunities, and life circumstances. A person is more likely to bounce back and stabilize permanently or temporarily at the refugee stage if he has received and enjoyed admiration for the 'valiant struggle,' or found a formula that appeals to his rigid sense of coherence (i.e., if he has 'accepted deafness' but on strictly limited terms). Antonovsky[38] suggested that positive coping does not result from wish-fulfilling fantasies ('There will be a cure one day.'), or emotional expression ('I feel bad today.'), or self-blame ('How did I get scarlet fever?' 'Why can't I lipread better?') All of these are likely to perpetuate the refugee state. An innate distaste for deaf people as one has always seen them would also impede progress; so would rejection by the local deaf community; and so would a belief that one's personal or economic survival depends on communicating in the old ways (i.e., orally). Finally, a slip-back is also more likely if there is a history of deference to the wishes of family members – or a belief that only family can help manage the interchange with the mainstream world.

The deafened person is *more likely* to move on to subsequent stages if her family and friends are willing to adapt to new ways of communicating. Also, if resources are available to help her absorb the shock – that is, if there are people to guide her through both the technical transition (the acquisition of assistive devices) and the social transition. These resources increase the manageability element of the sense of coherence. Antonovsky saw coping well as the capacity to incorporate relevant strategies and to change the nature of one's cognitions (i.e., ways of seeing the challenges). The likelihood of progress also increases if the deafened person is at a stage of life when she normally changes friends or becomes independent of family norms (e.g., is going off to college).

2.4.5 Deaf Activism: 'I Am Deaf, Dammit'

In the bereavement model, the stage that follows bargaining is depression. In the coming-out model, the stage that follows identity recognition is activism. (Cass referred to this as Identity Pride, based on the term 'gay pride.')

Our acquaintance with many deafened people supports *activism* rather than depression as the next stage for most people. Activism is an intensification of the consciousness we see in the identity recognition stage. Deafness becomes central to their identity, and they resist forces that would shut them out of events. Activism enables the individual to transfer the responsibility for difficulties from herself to an oppressive and inaccessible society.[39] The not-yet-ready person doubts whether the world is ready for deafness; in contrast, the deaf activist doesn't care if it's ready: no accommodation is unreasonable if it forces the hearing mainstream to deal with deafness. Through her actions, the deafened person is demanding that the hearing world work through the adjustment issues alongside her.

> My employer persisted in announcing required overtime over the public address system, and I decided to insist that they inform me in some accessible medium – perhaps face to face.

Day after day, I watched my co-workers stay for overtime, perhaps earning $70 a shift in extra income, while I stood my
ground. Meanwhile, my family persisted in passing messages
to me through each other: 'Tell him to come over.' 'Tell him to
call.' I refused to call back or acknowledge those messages.
After all, I had a TTY and they had my number. I knew my Deaf
friends happily let hearing people make calls to other hearing
people for them. I guess for them, efficiency was more important than pushing the issue. For me, making the effort to get a
TTY or use the relay service was more important than anything
they ever had to say. It was a statement of acceptance they
never made.

M.A.

Deafened people may become even more activist than people
who have always been deaf, because when they still had their
hearing they fully expected access, and the new inequities shock
them. They tell friends of their experiences, and their friends,
equally appalled, encourage them to complain. So they do complain, and it feels good – it feels as if they are taking control.
They may even achieve some change, which also feels good and
provides direct benefits such as access to academic, employment, and community opportunities. They join forces with other
deaf people and receive peer validation. Working on common
activism campaigns may help deafened people achieve acceptance from the deaf community – acceptance that was less forthcoming at the earlier stages. Thus the person who progresses
from identity recognition to activism is less likely to bounce back
into the refugee mode. A healthy amount of activism can have
professional benefits, because services for the deaf and hard of
hearing population need to be delivered and administered.
Deafened people may find that their insight into the hearing
world, in combination with their good speech, gives them an
unfair advantage over deaf people, especially if they can also
sign.

Activism helps immeasurably in accepting deafness, but there
are also some risks. One is that the activism will lead to separat-

I got my first taste of activism when I joined an accessibility task force. It shocked me when the deaf and hard-of-hearing members of that group were shunted off to subcommittees for their like kind, while the weighty issues of what kinds of access to advocate for were being discussed by the business leaders – hearing people. 'Consumer involvement' and 'cultural sensitivity' were a matter of lip service: ultimately, achieving public access was going to entail dealing with specific public places, yet that task was assigned to a committee full of hearing people. Of course, this approach made it unnecessary to provide interpreters and actually have to deal with the nuisance of deaf people's points of view. Before anyone had identified me as a deaf person, I'd had a seat at the table, and I wasn't going to start sitting at the kids' table letting adults make the decisions.

I've heard deaf people ask hearing people, 'Do you think we deaf people are capable of leadership?' Well, not if you have to ask permission, you're not! Sometimes I felt like I was pushing the hearing world with one arm and dragging the deaf world with the other.

K.W.

ism and to a complete rejection of the past 'hearing' life and values. A second is that the activism will consume all of life's other priorities. It may become a tool for deferring real acceptance, or identity synthesis; and it may serve to deflect criticisms that the individual is avoiding accepting deafness: 'How can I be avoiding deafness when it is all I think about and talk about every day?'

Deafened people who conceal their hearing past and become leaders and career deaf advocates may well be among those who have remained in this stage. In reference to the conventional wisdom that converts are often more observant than those born into a religion, we use the metaphor 'religious convert' for someone who lingers at this stage.

A number of deafened adolescents and young adults choose to attend deaf college and university programs. In response to the

Deaf Culture, which tends to dominate in these programs, the deafened student may give up and withdraw to the identity concession stage, in the hope of finding some other educational program; alternatively, she may become an activist. Some activists take up the banner of the Deaf cause and assimilate with their new fellows. Other activists – those with stronger nerve and a larger appetite for conflict – take up the deafened cause, remaining in the Deaf Culture while advocating for their own inclusion in that world. Either approach fits into the model at this step.

Progression beyond this stage may depend on the reactions of others. If they are negative – that is, if others continue to disparage deafness as a viable alternative identity – this may reinforce the deafened person's need for activism, and identity foreclosure may occur.

2.4.6 Depression

In the bereavement model, depression precedes acceptance. It is the phase during which the bereaved person gives in to the situation. The letting go of the quest for control has been called the indication that 'acceptance' has occurred.[40] The depression stage is absent from Cass's coming-out model, which progresses directly from activism (pride) to acceptance (synthesis) if activism is unexpectedly met with acceptance by others. We believe that depression is a valid stage in the process of accepting deafness, although activism precedes depression.[41] There can be depression throughout the adjustment process, especially among people who have limited resilience. However, at each earlier stage the identity is 'more like' one of the other stages we have described.

> One day I heard a sound: it was the sound of my own life crashing ... As I sat pondering the wreckage, I saw the paradox. There I was, being so tremendously self-aware with self-help training and all, that I hadn't seen myself being sucked up into this consuming activism. But when I collapsed, blubbering, in the shower, I knew it meant something. I had quit my job to

study for a PhD; I'd prepared so well for it that I fully expected to complete in the minimum time. After deferring academic milestones for four years because 'ALDA needed me' to do this or that, the endless pressure to keep less and less for myself finally took its toll.

K.W.

The end of the activism stage may be marked by an abrupt crash and stage of depression as the individual realizes that no amount of activism will ever change all the wrongs in society. The depression may be simply a 'reality check,' or reconciliation, and not take the form of clinical depression. If the person has received considerable positive feedback for his deaf-activist views, it may simply be an episode of burnout. Those who remain in the activist stage may never experience that let-down or depression. In depression, the individual stops enjoying the things he used to enjoy. The satisfactions of a rousing campaign of activism are lost. The prospect of socializing, whether with deaf or hearing people, may become uninviting. Hopes for the future may be relinquished, not specifically because of fear of coping with deafness but rather as part of a general malaise. Perhaps the time and energy required to accept deafness have been at the expense of other personal and career priorities.

A stage of depression may be the marker of the onset of true acceptance.

In ALDA, I got involved in activism, tried to participate in leadership activities, and essentially tried to attain that self-actualization that I'd been missing in the 'outside world.' From the shared experience of ALDA people, I concluded that it was people's lack of understanding that had limited me. Now that I was 'home,' I would be the person I could be. After a couple of years of involvement, I grew frustrated and disillusioned. Being deaf didn't bother anyone, but my socioeconomic status and the education I never had seemed to disqualify me.

> Depressed, I killed my pain with marathon training, and almost quit ALDA. I came for the last time, to say goodbye. Instead, I adjusted my expectations and reduced my role.
>
> M.A.

2.4.7 Identity Synthesis: Accepting Deafness

In this final stage, deafness becomes less central to the deafened person's identity. The person is still deaf, but is no longer isolated, as she has acquired friends who are deaf or who can communicate. Deafness has integrated itself with her core identity and social environment. Although she may still support activist movements for the betterment of the deaf community, much of her fervour has subsided as she refocuses on enriching holistic aspects in her life.

> I regret what it has cost me professionally to spend so much of the past ten years dealing with my deafness. I enjoy being a cultural interpreter, helping hearing people understand deafness a little better and giving encouragement to deafened people who are still dealing with their issues. But I'm also eager to do *my* things – the things I was doing before, that I would have kept doing if I weren't deaf, that had nothing to do with deafness. I know I need to invest a little activism to make sure I get the accommodations I need in order to have a fair chance, but I'm worn out from doing it all day, every day. I want some peace.
>
> K.W.

We use the metaphor 'immigrant' for this stage. Mindful of the old country but established in the new one, the deafened person can now refocus on personal development and return to the quest for self-actualization. A person who has attained identity synthesis, or acceptance, feels less compelled to get intensely involved in the social, self-help, and political issues of late deafness. He

TABLE 2.2
Model of deafened adjustment and comparative models

Model of deafened adjustment	Comparison to:	
	Coming out (Cass)	Bereavement (Kübler-Ross)
Identity confusion	Identity confusion	Denial
Identity comparison	Identity comparison	Anger (why me?)
Identity concession	Identity tolerance	Bargaining
Identity recognition	Identity acceptance	
Deaf activism	Identity pride	
Depression		Depression
Identity synthesis	Identity synthesis	Acceptance

may continue to seek out deafened groups for socializing, or for self-actualization, or for self-help when there are specific, isolated issues of conflict with the hearing mainstream. Otherwise, the deaf identity takes its place within the whole person, which also accommodates the family, career, and other interests. This compartmentalization counteracts the nature of activism, through which deafness may 'spread' to consume the entire identity.[42]

For the disability to stop being central to one's self-concept requires 'fashioning an alternative identity based on strengths.'[43] In this process, the disability is not denied; rather, the person deals with it by seeking appropriate help. This reorientation is achieved after years of experience with the disability. Possibly, the attitudes in some groups work against the achievement of synthesis, by obligating or compelling people to remain 'active' members and by inciting continued militancy beyond a degree that is helpful in personal terms.

2.5 Comparison

Table 2.2 compares the Model of Deafened Adjustment with the 'coming out' model and the bereavement model.

Chapter 3

Effect on Relationships

As was the case in the previous chapter, much of this chapter's discussion of the effects of deafness on relationships refers to Goffman's work on stigma. The discussion of passing, disclosing, covering, and relations with other deaf people often needs only to paraphrase the principles thoroughly described by Goffman.

3.1 Inconvenience and Stigma

Several of the common responses to deaf people from family, friends, acquaintances, and strangers resemble those made to many other stigmatized groups.[1] One is the well-meaning inquiry into the etiology or management of the condition; another is admiring remarks about deaf people, or sympathy with their 'plight.' People try to demonstrate their open-mindedness out of a desire not to seem prejudiced. A similar overreaction is for people to recognize and extol the deaf person's achievements, proclaiming them noteworthy or even surprising even though they are not. This gives the deaf person the impression that people are patronizing. Also, it is too easy for them to infer that the general public expects very little from them.

Approaches to communication with other people are strongly influenced by perceptions of their entire group. People often speak in ways that precisely fit their expectations of their interaction partner – but their expectations may be inappropriate. When

Common Questions

Why do you have good speech? My neighbour's nephew is
    deaf and even his parents can't understand him.
Is sign language universal? Why not?
Can you remember sounds and music?
Can you hear your own voice?
Can you lipread?
Can you drive?
How will your daughter learn to talk?
Can you read Braille? (We wish we were kidding.)

disabled people are perceived as dependent and helpless, they
may be seen, treated, and addressed as children. A common style
of communication when nondisabled people encounter people
with disabilities is for the former to select an inappropriate register for communication, such as baby talk or talking a-b-n-o-r-m-
a-l-l-y s-l-o-w-l-y. Also, if someone has concluded that people
with hearing loss tend to be less educated than hearing people,
interaction with any deaf person will trigger a simplified
approach. On meeting a disabled person who disproves the
expectation, and equals or outperforms him, a nondisabled person may perceive a serious threat to self-esteem.[2]

New acquaintances invariably compliment my speech – not as
in 'you gave a good speech' but as in 'you have good speech.'
If I want feedback on my lecture, I don't tell the audience that
I'm deaf. People are so fixated on my vocabulary and my pronunciation that I wonder if they are even listening to what I say.
                                                                    K.W.

3.1.1 Family

Social support plays an important role in coping with late deafness, as it does in any transition. Healthy relationships and a supportive social environment help balance out stress and thereby limit the negative impact of deafness. Psychosocial support speeds recovery from almost any medical condition. Indeed, social integration (versus isolation) has as strong an effect on all-cause, age-adjusted mortality as smoking or cholesterol levels.[3]

In a crisis, most people can usually turn to their family as the prime social support network. This is not necessarily true in the case of deafened people. Family and friends often have as many problems with deafness as deafened people themselves do. According to deafened people, deafness limits conversation within the family and causes strain and irritation; also, other family members often don't have the time or the patience to keep repeating until the deafened person comprehends. Nevertheless, deafened people often describe their family and friends as sympathetic even while impatient. Deafened people are more likely to describe their family as unsupportive; they often observe that friends are more willing to make adjustments. Even compared with hard-of-hearing people, people with hearing loss over 70 dB (severe hearing loss) are significantly more likely to be separated or divorced or to report their marriage has suffered.[4]

Families often decide (by default) to cope with a family member's deafness by pretending the condition does not exist. Thomas Edison's Christmas Day celebrations with his young children were described this way:

> When the children were young they began the day by waking their parents. With their uncle, they played the phonograph in the second floor hall, gathered their stockings from the fireplace in the Living Room, and sang carols outside of their mother and father's room. After singing, they went in and sat on the bed. Theodore [Edison's son] noted that '... I think father got very little out of it, because of course he couldn't hear, and having all these kids climbing all over the place and looking at these presents didn't mean much to him. But it was wonderful for us.' This ritual was followed by opening larger gifts under the tree.[5]

There is no indication in this that there was anything unacceptable about 'Father getting very little out of it.' The typical family acts as if embarrassing the deafened person by noticing his deafness would be worse than cutting him off by ignoring it. This behaviour seems to confirm the deafened person's fear that even his own family has stigmatized him.

Misunderstandings about the effectiveness of lipreading and the benefits of hearing aids commonly interfere with interactions between deafened people and their families. The family believes, and often instructs others, that the deafened person 'can understand you if you look straight at her when you talk.' Actually, lipreading is of limited benefit to many who attempt it, yet almost anyone can lipread the standard 'test questions' using only rudimentary guessing, because 99 per cent of the time, the sentence after 'Can you lipread?' is 'What am I saying?' This just encourages people to think things are fine. (Experienced lipreaders often say the best response to 'Can you read lips?' is 'Oh, hit or miss, depends on the speaker.' The wags say the best response is 'No!')

> Despite the close contact of marriage, my ex-husband admits he had no idea that I had any difficulty with lipreading – that it exhausted me and that half the time I didn't have a clue what he was saying. He had persuaded himself that my encouragement of signed communication was an overreaction, a mere romantic adventure in Deaf Land on my part, and one that I would eventually get over and return to normal. Actually, I was barely hanging on, and my sign language classes were a life preserver in a rapidly rising tide.
>
> K.W.

Family members may think that hearing aids restore hearing the same way that eyeglasses correct visual anomalies. They don't realize that the sound quality often leaves a great deal to be desired, and that with severe and profound deafness the sound perception is often at best adequate to capture the rhythms of speech. Family pressure, more than internal motivation, pushes many people to investigate hearing aids or a cochlear implant.

Family 'encouragement' – to 'not give up,' to 'try harder,' to 'never say can't,' and so on – is fundamentally self-serving, in that it obviates the significant adjustments that a transition to (for example) sign language would require from them. Deafened people report feeling frustrated, impatient, and even angry at the perceived insensitivity of their families;[6] even so, they are vulnerable to this 'encouragement.' Most people want to retain the love and support of their families, and perceive that love and support as being conditional on living up to the preferences their families convey so guilefully.

> My family could not bother to learn the fingerspelling alphabet in the twenty years since I became deaf. Yet they could barely avoid tripping over one another in the race to the telephone to call the cochlear implant clinic to set up an appointment for me.
>
> M.A.

A deafened person has little control over communication modes unless other family members make a mutual effort with them. It hardly ever happens. This lack of support reflects the approach to hearing loss encountered in the medical profession, which considers that the person suffers deafness, not the family, and which centres rehabilitation on the deaf individual. We must recognize that late deafness is a *social* disability. In compensation for this deficit in family support, many deafened people who are members of ALDA refer spontaneously to that group as their 'family,' or 'tribe,' or 'home.'

> One of the most enduring principles of ALDA is that there is no 'right' way to communicate and that any effective medium is

legitimate. This principle obliges people to stand on their head and blink Morse code if that is what it takes. A person who has a very limited ability to communicate will feel much less pressured, inadequate, and insecure in this environment than, say, at the family dinner table, where a certain type and standard of communication has likely been imposed.

In each issue, the ALDA newsletter has published an interview in which a member answers a standard set of self-disclosure questions. One of the questions used to be, 'When did you accept your deafness?' Before the establishment of the annual ALDA convention, which brought large numbers of deafened adults together for mutual support, interviewees described acceptance in terms of objective, practical necessity. Examples: 'My audiologist told me to accept it.' 'My hearing aid wasn't enough any more.' 'I was referred for a cochlear implant.' 'I haven't accepted it.'[7] In contrast, in more than two-thirds of the interviews published between 1990 and 1994 – after ALDA emerged as an alternative social outlet on a national level – interviewees referred to acceptance mainly in terms of social interactions: 'I found people who cared.' 'I realized I was not alone.' With or without ALDA's encouragement, the people who have experienced the group's social support network have completely redefined for themselves the entire concept of 'accepting deafness.' People used to conclude that they had accepted deafness once they had acknowledged the permanence of their auditory failure; now it seems that they define acceptance as the feeling of being accepted by others. It also appears that the type of acceptance desired most is the kind provided within groups of deafened people – that is, uncritical and understanding acceptance of whatever the communication modes will be.

3.1.2 Friends and Acquaintances

Deafened people are more likely to have no friends and difficulty making friends, even compared to people with hearing losses of lesser severity.[8] Friends and acquaintances perceive a personality change because personality is reflected in how communication occurs, and deafness has altered the old channels. As with any stigma, people feel uncomfortable, and afraid of using words that may offend. Thus, they avoid mentioning deafness, and they monitor what they say to avoid expressions such as 'Did you hear that ...' and 'I'll keep my ears open for ...' Some former friends may not co-operate with the effort required for communication. Finally, they may feel awkward, or threatened or repelled by the intense feelings the deafened person may express during the adjustment process.

> Communication in relationships is difficult enough without having to work at the mechanics of it. Once I realized I had options, I wanted new friends to be able to accommodate that. I wasn't interested in dating anyone who didn't sign and expected me to lipread. I found it amusing and annoying when I would say to a guy, 'I'm deaf, I sign,' and he would respond, 'Oh, that's all right.' As in, 'I don't mind.' Maybe I mind that he isn't and he doesn't.
>
> K.W.

Disidentifiers are symbols that are associated with the absence of the stigma and that make others doubt whether the perceived stigma fully applies. A prestigious job can be a disidentifier; in this case, one would expect people to make more allowances for a deaf doctor than for a deaf student or a deaf file clerk. In the general population, members of privileged classes, genders, and ethnic groups tend to suffer less from stigmas.

3.2 The Purpose of Communication

Communication serves two purposes: to *convey information* and to *foster relationships*. When people help deafened people by writing down important points on a notepad, they are conveying content and helping alleviate barriers to the exchange of information. Deafened people are grateful to family and friends who offer this type of assistance. By the same token, when people refuse to repeat the last three sentences of a shaggy dog story while the rest of the group is doubled over in laughter, they typically say something like, 'It wasn't that important,' or 'You had to be there,' or 'I'll tell you later.' Deafened people invariably mention such statements as sore points in their relationships with family and friends. Too often, people respect the *information* purpose of communication while not recognizing the *relationship* purpose.[9]

In relationships, the main dimensions of communication are dominance (or submission) and affiliation.[10] Hearing ability usually allows hearing people to dominate. Being consigned involuntarily to the submissive role can make the deafened person feel disaffiliated. Frequent loss of content and insensitive repair can have the same effect. The relational goals of communication – to convey inclusion, control, or affection – can all be jeopardized. The use of communicative acts to fulfil relationship needs is obvious in several practices that might seem peculiar from the perspective of 'communication = content.' For example, people with progressive loss often continue to use the telephone long past the point where they can understand any words, just to hear the sound of another person's voice. Elderly people with hearing loss may converse by alternating lengthy active and passive stretches, each just maintaining the other's monologue. This pattern minimizes the impact of not fully comprehending each other, and respects the relational ritual of communication.[11]

Too often, people simply fail to respect the importance of chit-chat and inconsequential dialogue. As a result, their idea of adequate communication access results in a reduced quality of life. 'It may be said that I was shut off from that particular kind of social intercourse which is small talk. I am glad of it ... I have no doubt that my nerves are stronger and better today than they would have been if I had heard all the foolish conversation and other meaningless sounds that normal people hear.'[12] Thomas Edison is sometimes described as 'well adjusted' for that passage. An alternative explanation is that he was exceptionally cold, or had thoroughly rationalized his situation to the point where he no longer felt he deserved or even wanted warm human relationships. The tone of the quote sounds a lot like, 'Stupid cake. I didn't want any. It was probably stale anyway, and it would just have gone straight to my hips.'

As a result of many years of passing for hearing, I had no close friends at the time of my first marriage, and had a civil ceremony mainly because there would have been no one to invite to an actual wedding. I rationalized that wedding celebrations were a waste of time, energy, and money. Mentally I ridiculed colleagues who were preparing or reflecting upon their 'whole nine yards' of satin and lace. Yet every time a wedding party passed my house in a cacaphony of horns, I would regret that I had not had *my* day.

K.W.

We grant that social interaction has different degrees of importance to different people. Some people are extroverted; others are introverted. Some already have all the friends they feel they need; others are still building their network of relationships. However, even the exchange of meaningless courtesies with strangers is an important part of living a civil existence and feeling worthwhile. Scorning that sort of communication as unimportant – primarily because one can't do it – is the ultimate devaluation of one's social worth.

When I was hospitalized recovering from the meningitis that deafened me, I had no way to communicate with anyone. While other patients could chat with roommates and cleaning staff to pass the time and keep the spirits up, I could not. Granted, I got the same food, water, and medication that any other comparable patient received, but I received none of the social support because no one considered chit-chat as being worth the effort.

M.A.

Some people have asserted incorrectly that 'deafened adults do not learn to sign.' We have seen many deafened adults signing with pleasure at deafened gatherings, where they are free from criticism by deaf people ('You don't sign well.') and hearing people ('Why are you signing? You could try to lipread me.'). The calibre of the *signing* may be poor, but the *communication* is excellent. The strong relationships that develop are evidence of the importance in communication of eye contact and mutual effort. We like sign communication because it enables people to maintain eye contact, which is central to the relationship part of communication, without sacrificing any content. We choose to strive for proper sign language, but we don't think it's critical. It would be effective as long as all of the communicators to use the same sign language, linguistically referred to as 'home signs.' For families with elderly people who are convinced they are unable to learn sign language, we often suggest letting the elders devise the signs and what they will mean; the junior family members can then learn to use that vocabulary. However, we know people who took up sign language successfully after retirement, and recommend not making any hasty, age-based conclusions.

On the old game show *Password*, one person had a hidden word and had to give one- or two-word clues to the other person, who was to guess what the hidden 'password' was. There was once an episode in which a team of two men was given the password 'podiatrist.' The clue-giver offered, 'baby doctor.' With no hesitation whatsoever, the password guesser answered 'podiatrist,' which proves that you don't have to use the correct words, just words that mean what your communication partner thinks they mean. And so it is with proper sign language, versus home signs.

Some semblance of 'proper' sign language can open up one's social windows to a whole new set of people, but only the deafened person himself can decide which population he wants to communicate with. Some will always advise a newly deafened person against sign language, saying, 'But who will you sign with? Your family and friends can't sign. You'll be limiting yourself to a small group of people who can sign.' According to the Deaf Census figures cited earlier, almost 1 per cent of the population is deaf. Including hearing people who sign, American Sign Language is the fourth most used language in the United States,[13] just as British Sign Language is the fourth most used language in Britain.[14] People tend to associate with those who make them feel most comfortable, whether that is fellow bodybuilders, feminists, or Orthodox Jews, so there is nothing intrinsically peculiar about someone deciding to socialize mainly with fellow deaf or deafened people. Most people would consider themselves to have plenty of friends long before making the acquaintance of 1 per cent of the population. Seeking friends within a specific circle does not preclude maintaining ties to the broader community. In fact, acquiring an additional mode of communication *increases* rather than decreases one's ability to find comfortable social relationships. The only people who do not benefit from this are those who *become* the less comfortable social circle.

3.3 Passing

Because of the reactions of hearing people, the desire to conceal one's deafness is all too rational – sometimes it is even necessary. While a deafened person may not think explicitly in terms of 'stigma,' she knows that social encounters will be awkward. It can harm a relationship to inform the other person of your hearing loss, if it makes him feel awkward. Unfortunately, that relationship can also be harmed if you *don't* inform him and he finds out later, when he is likely to be offended that you didn't trust him with the information in the first place. Candor may require sharing more information than the situation warrants. Say, for instance, that you want to buy gloves. The options are (a) to stride into the accessories department and state, 'I am deaf and I would like to buy a pair of kidskin gloves, size 7,' or (b) to be forced to apologize later for mishearing and not having warned the saleslady not to speak with her head inside the cupboard.

On the eve of a conference, I went to dinner at a restaurant with my then-husband and a man with a strong accent. In the dim light and with clanking dishes all around us, I smiled, nodded, and generally did my impression of the gracious spouse. When I spoke at the conference over which this man presided, I disclosed my hearing loss as part of my presentation. Later, he approached me to object that I hadn't given him the opportunity to speak differently so that I could understand him better. He felt slighted – evidently I hadn't thought his conversation was worth the extra effort to comprehend. I had passed, all right, but in passing I had insulted the other party. Personally, I doubt whether the man could have done anything to enable me to comprehend better, what with his accent, the lighting, and the noise. The only relevance the meeting had for me was that it was a restaurant and I was hungry. Had I brought my deafness to his attention, facilitating my comprehension would have superseded the main object of the meeting, where I was merely a social participant. I don't suppose it would have consoled him that I hadn't understood my husband either.

K.W.

A practical reason for attempting to pass for hearing is that the co-operation of others is no guarantee of success. Even when the other person is willing to take a stab at viewing the deafness as merely a difference among equals, after the second or third unsuccessful try at transmitting a particular message, he feels heightened anxiety about this unwelcome responsibility because he does not know what to do other than smile awkwardly, rationalize that it wasn't important anyway, and give up. On some level, he resents the deaf person for having made him feel inadequate to the task.

I am still not convinced that attempting to pass is a bad thing, if it has a chance of success, but it has adverse effects if it doesn't work. My undergraduate classmates later told me they thought I was an utter snob throughout the first year, in the front row with my back to the class, attentive only to the professor. My lack of interaction and reaction was especially conspicuous because I was one of only four women in the class. I passed in the sense that they didn't realize I couldn't hear them, but they didn't think I was normal, and they initially treated me not as a person who cannot hear but as a person who doesn't respond to friendly overtures. Once I began to sit sideways, I was able to develop a bit more rapport and co-operation with my classmates – essentially to survive academically in that program – without giving up the proximity I needed in order to lipread. But a professor once told me that if I died before he did, he would bury me on my side.

K.W.

Attempting to pass for hearing is appealing because others behave naturally if they believe they are interacting with someone like themselves and not a stigmatized person. On the other hand, when the deaf person attempts to pass for hearing, he is precluded from using modified communication techniques that require the co-operation of the other person. Passing sacrifices the *content* of the communication for the sake of its *relationship* aspects. According to Goffman, attempts to pass transform social situations into information management challenges, in that they aim to prevent those who 'shouldn't know' from discovering the condition. Two common techniques are faked comprehension and monopolizing the conversation (to obviate listening). These techniques are flawed: regarding the first, a failure to guess correctly will lead to an inappropriate response; regarding the second, people will become annoyed at the incessant prattle. Passing can be facilitated by intimates who *do* know and can help carry out the masquerade. Many spouses fill the role of covering for the deafened partner by repeating, answering for them, and camouflaging mistakes.

Most deafened people develop stock responses for passing situations. Often used are neutral comments – 'That's interesting,' 'I'm not sure,' – combined with a pleasant expression. Ideally, the other person has provided some clue with his own expression so that the response can be customized a little: 'Oh!' with a sympathetic look if it seems bad, or 'That's nice,' and a smile if it looks good. Sarcasm and teasing are deadly to the passer.

When the attempt to conceal the hearing loss is unsuccessful, the deafened person ends up seeming gauche, snobbish, inattentive, wooden, and distant. This can hurt others' feelings if they have tried to be friendly. The only remedy to this is to disclose the condition and throw oneself at their mercy. But doing so doubles the stigma, because in addition to being deaf, one is also showing oneself to be dishonest. The only sure way to prevent disclosure is social isolation.

Generally, I wasn't very effective at passing. I would go to clubs to meet people, and never get far in conversations. My best memory was a costume event when I dressed in a gorilla suit, acted like a gorilla, and made only gorilla talk all night. I was able to be the 'funny guy' and enjoy attention that I never otherwise used to get. No one figured I was deaf – a weird guy who doesn't know when a joke has gotten old, perhaps, but not deaf. I recall it as a great night out, sad as it seems now.

M.A.

3.4 Disclosing

Disclosure can occur involuntarily in a variety of ways. There may be an embarrassing incident such that the only alternative is to explain that deafness was the cause. Someone who knows the truth and perhaps doesn't realize that others don't know may disclose it. Someone else may wield the secret for the power it gives him or her to disclose it at will. Finally, a person who has lived with a deaf person (often a family member) may notice the signs of lipreading and faking.

It wasn't a deliberate disclosure in the sense of militancy or maturity, but I once disclosed my deafness in the act of changing a hearing aid battery. I had been carrying on a daily bus stop relationship for some months with a young woman I thought I could get to know better. I had never mentioned my deafness, blaming occasional requests for repetition on the traffic noise. One day, my battery died in the middle of her sentence. By then our chats had grown comfortable enough that I didn't perceive it as a big risk to change my battery in front of her. After I did, and replaced the aid, she asked, 'What was that?' I replied that it was my hearing aid. Her expression changed, and our conversation was cut off abruptly when a bus arrived and she jumped on without a word. I realized in a moment that it wasn't her bus. She was never at that stop again.

M.A.

After laboriously trying to pass, the individual may decide to stop trying to pass and to force the world to accept him. In more practical terms, the person may come to realize that his mistakes have become too frequent or serious and that the choice is not between stigma and no stigma, but between the stigma of deafness and the stigma of cluelessness. Pauline Ashley, wife of British MP Jack Ashley, said the issue is not how to hide the deafness but rather how to minimize its consequences.[15] The individual must go on to unlearn the art of concealment. The decision to stop trying to pass is typically seen as the mark of maturity and acceptance.

Voluntary disclosure can be achieved through the use of 'stigma symbols,' purposeful slips, behaviours, and verbal disclosures. 'Stigma symbols' include conspicuous hearing aids, signing in public, giving a telephone number with a TTY suffix, bringing an interpreter to a function, or displaying a lapel button or card bearing an inscription such as 'lipreader: please speak clearly.' Without anything being said, the observer realizes that these symbols denote deafness. Purposeful slips include requesting repetition or notes when the message may have been obviously unimportant or easy to guess, or perhaps accentuating deaf enunciation when the deaf person has perfect speech. Associating with other deaf people is a behaviour that may send a message that one is deaf. The *signs* of deafness (for instance, mistakes) cause annoyance in others; *symbols* such as buttons or cards tend to cause others to be kind, but patronizing.[16]

> The historical concealment of deafness may explain why the mainstream population often cannot recognize its stigma symbols. When I wore red behind-the-ear hearing aids framed against my fair skin by my dark hair in a ponytail, I actually received compliments (from behind my back, naturally) on the ornaments on my sunglasses. People have sought me out for conversations during breaks in meetings when the interpreter has slipped out to the ladies' room. I suspect they think it is the interpreter who is deaf, because *she* is the one who is signing. I just sit there looking 'normal.'
>
> K.W.

Verbal disclosure, seemingly the simplest method, must follow 'disclosure etiquette.' Even though honesty demands disclosure, custom is that we do not talk about ourselves without invitation. Disclosure etiquette requires that the fact be somehow worked into the conversation (e.g., 'Being deaf, I find that ...'). Unfortunately, deafness is not always pertinent to the topic of conversation, which leaves a choice between symbols, slips, and behaviours, or announcements about oneself. The latter elicits the reaction, 'How nice for you. Thank you for sharing,' more often than a behavioural change to make communication easier. This is likely because the disclosure does not provide any guidance on how to proceed, other than to make allowances for mistakes. Scholars have suggested that disabled people can improve social interaction by putting nondisabled people at ease through matter-of-fact guidance in successful strategies for coping. However, amending the disclosure to incorporate sufficient guidance would greatly increase the conspicuity of the announcement, and that would violate the etiquette rule of not dominating the proceedings with self-centred concerns.

Even after disclosure, there is still pressure to 'cover.' Covering consists of behaviours similar to passing, except that the purpose is not to keep the stigma secret, but rather to minimize the degree to which the condition becomes the centre of attention. The stigmatized person must restrict the display of failings to those central to her condition, and generally act as 'normal' as possible. This requires her to organize social situations in such a way as to minimize the impact. For this, the strategies and tactics can be elaborate.[17]

I have not skimped on disclosure. I have written guidelines on conference access that have been adopted by my professional colleagues and that include clear protocols for offering and booking interpreters. I have explained the scarcity of interpreters and the need to book early, and furnished lists of interpreters. I have explained how certain situations call for team interpreting. I have checked up after the requests, just to be safe – and have rarely found things under control. Typically, after sitting on my request for six weeks, with two weeks to go, the organizers return to me and say, 'Would you make the arrangements? This is just so complicated.' (If you think booking interpreters is complicated, try being deaf.)

And I don't think it is entirely about putting them at ease. I have openly talked about deafness, putting it in their scientific context. They feel at ease enough to ask me if I couldn't just come early (so as not disturb others) and sit in the front row, and maybe wear an FM system, because it would be cheaper. They are so focused on the cost to themselves – this little eight

> or sixteen hours' worth of interpreting and disturbance, every
> couple of years – their minor share of the cost I bear twenty-
> four hours a day, seven days a week, that fundamental human
> rights says should be shared.
>
> K.W.

The pressure to 'cover' is also a symptom of tokenism, although tokenism may not have been intended. In tokenism, the group openly wants a member of a particular group, but they actually want a person who closely resembles a middle-aged, white, right-handed, able-bodied, Protestant, heterosexual, male captain of industry. A token-seeking group breathes a sigh of relief when it is able to recruit a person with a mild hearing loss to stand in for the deaf and hard-of-hearing population. Another group may have no desire for a token – it may not care one way or the other about deafness, or it may be motivated by the genuine desire to expand diversity – but may still prefer that the individual cover, because reminders seem to be irrelevant distractions or bids for attention.

In most group situations, disclosure provides little direct benefit. It can help avoid the dishonesty stigma, as well as misunderstandings about the reason for mistakes or withdrawal. However, the empathy that individual members have for the deafened person's difficulties cannot usually overcome the chaos that most group interactions become. Alternatively, the self-discipline required to accommodate the deafened person may put a damper on the group. For instance, if the chair insists that everyone face the deafened person, the participants may co-operate but the discussion may become stilted. In many settings, the group merely barrels on. Groups tend to be most grateful if the deafened person acts as if included while making few demands for *actual* inclusion. The worst situation of all is when the deafened person becomes a 'mascot' for the group; here, the group acknowledges the condition, and thus indicates that the deaf person isn't stigmatized, but its actions indicate otherwise.

At my farewell party, my colleagues and friends donned surgical masks, greatly amusing themselves. They though this was funny, and from their perspective I can appreciate that it was. They had been fairly co-operative with repetition for me, and I had been quite facile with both lipreading and covering. To single this out for special treatment at my luncheon was to state the unstated – that it had been conspicuous all along, merely humoured, through conscious efforts that never became natural to the point of not noticing. I had endeared myself to them much like the family dog – welcome at the table, but all the same, still a dog.

K.W.

3.5 Making New Friends in the Deaf Community

As a former member of the mainstream society, the deafened person likely feels little affiliation with other deaf people. After being a member of the hearing world, she would rather remain isolated on its periphery than united in a deafened world. 'If people with poor eyesight or warts do not identify with one another, why should those with poor hearing?'[18] 'They' have a stigma.

Stigmatized people begin their relations with the group with ambivalence.[19] Being affiliated with a group one finds repulsive is a source of shame. At first, discrediting the affiliation is easier than overcoming the repulsion. Over time, the individual experiences cycles of approaching and distancing, which are often linked to other changes in life status. There may come a turning point where she recognizes the affiliation – for example, she may realize that her hearing friends view her deaf friends as 'freaks,' though she had never seen them that way. The turning point may occur during a period of introspection, such as hospitalization.

I have never sat still for discrimination. I have objected more than a few times to slights that other deaf people have accepted. But I have found myself impatient with artificial issues created just for the sake of militancy. I recall a huge fuss being raised in the workplace over a perfectly adequate inter- preter, the holder of a degree in interpreting and the child of deaf parents, who had just not scraped together the money and experience to take and pass the certification exams. Bear- ing in mind that she was interpreting employee training and low-priority department meetings and not discipline or arbitra- tion matters, I just couldn't support the deaf employee's griev- ance. It annoyed me to be caught in the middle and expected to help the the grievor play the system just because I was deaf too.

M.A.

The success of deafened people's contact with the local deaf community can vary widely. The acquisition of signing skills does not occur as rapidly as most hearing losses, and too often this leaves deafened people with a gap between needs and abil- ity. In communities where Deaf people shun or ridicule those who sign poorly or who didn't attend the right deaf residential school, deafened people experience rejection. Whether or not it is the Deaf Culture's intention to leave deafened people bleed- ing on the sidewalk outside the deaf club (figuratively), that is the frequent emotional consequence. As long as those who sign poorly are discouraged from going places where their signing skills can improve, many late-deafened people will continue to struggle with sign language. This conspicuous struggle has led to claims that late-deafened people do not learn to sign.

I had been deaf for perhaps eight years without meeting any deaf people. A new counsellor at the vocational rehabilitation agency suggested I go to the deaf club. For six months, I kept the slip of paper with the address, but didn't do anything. Then I was riding a bus and saw three deaf people chatting easily with one another in sign language. When they got off, I noticed it was in front of the club. Three weeks later, in the middle of a particularly isolating night out at a music nightclub, I took the bus over to the deaf club, armed only with my fingerspelling alphabet. Even though I didn't talk to many people, I wasn't any more shut out than I had been at my usual clubs. I felt much more belonging than I felt among hearing people. I could understand a bit between fingerspelling and intuition. I thought, 'This is cool.'

M.A.

Those who learn sign language skills more readily can immerse themselves fully in Deaf Culture and hope to pass for Deaf. It is not the place of this book to 'out' anyone, but many recent and current Deaf leaders were also deafened later than early childhood, remember the auditory world, and benefit from the years they spent absorbing Hearing customs and values. Only recently have some deafened people begun to admit that they had previously been hearing, and even enjoyed music, although they accepted sign language as their adopted language and considered themselves deaf. The rejection of those 'not Deaf enough' has extended to late-deafened Gallaudet University President I. King Jordan, whose joyous appointment was followed quickly by complaints that a born-deaf president should have been selected. However, this discrimination seems to apply only to living deafened people. Many people held out as distinguished historical deaf figures were in fact late-deafened, including Beethoven, Edison, and Juliette Gordon Low. Of the first twenty-three presidents of the NAD (the U.S. National Association of the Deaf), twelve were deafened at age ten or later. Three were deafened at age 15, 16, and 18.[20]

Even after the affiliation is internalized, the individual may still feel ambivalent at the sight of others behaving in stereotyped ways and demonstrating the negative attributes that come with the stigma. As well, the individual can become bored with the group's propensity to interpret absolutely everything in terms of the condition: deaf Miss America, deaf Olympians, deaf actresses, deaf professional athletes, deaf inventors, and deaf politicians are interesting to the group foremost because they are deaf and only secondarily because of their other qualities. Not long ago, a deaf Internet discussion list[21] revealed the momentous cultural tidbit that Che Guevara was unable to dance because he was tone deaf. This illustrates two common traits of this cultural behaviour: claiming deaf 'ownership' of notable figures, however tenuous; and misunderstanding English idioms, in that *tone* deafness' has absolutely nothing at all to do with deafness either culturally or audiometrically.

Affiliation with the group enables the individual to see humour in the weaknesses of the stereotype while enjoying the folktales, which typically involve the stereotyped character triumphing over the 'normals.' Deaf humour is rife with these tales.

A deaf guy, a Russian, and a Cuban are riding on a train. The Russian opens a bottle of vodka, takes a drink, and throws the rest of the bottle out the window. The Cuban says, 'Why did you throw away all that vodka?' The Russian says, 'Where I come from, we have so much vodka, we are swimming in it.' Some miles later, the Cuban takes a big cigar out of his pocket, lights it, puffs once on it, and throws it out the window. The deaf guy asks, 'Why did you throw that whole cigar out the window?' The Cuban says, 'Oh, in Cuba we have so many cigars, we would never be able to smoke them all.' He sits, and he's thinking and thinking about all this, and then the deaf guy stands up and grabs the sleeping car porter, and throws him out the window. The Russian says, 'Why did you throw him out the window?!!' The deaf guy says, 'Where I come from, we have too many hearing people.'

A little hearing boy has a deaf uncle in an otherwise all-hearing family. One day, he takes his chewing gum and sticks it in his ears, like the earmolds of his uncle's hearing aids, and he says to his mother, 'Hey look, mom! I'm deaf!' His mother slaps him, and says, 'Go show your father.' The boy finds his father in the workshop and says, 'Look dad, I'm deaf!' His father raises his hand and slaps him hard on the face. 'You say that to your grandmother!' So the boy looks for the grandmother, who is now with the mother in the kitchen. 'Look Grandma, I'm deaf!' And the grandmother slaps him too. His mother says, 'Have you learned anything, son?' And the boy replies, 'I sure have. I've only been deaf for twenty minutes, and already I hate hearing people.'

Beyond simple affiliation lies the territory of activism, which involves a given group confronting mainstream society about the injustice of being stigmatized. The acceptance does not happen at the pace set by the activist. As time passes, others will reap the benefits of successful activism; in the meantime, the activist's own life tends to become even more different from normal. A stigma loses force gradually, typically by discussion through humour, and by more frequent encounters between the stigmatized people and 'normals' until the differences no longer cause awkwardness. For example, divorce is no longer stigmatized, nor is Irish ethnicity.

People who are a little more vocal and a little more connected can end up being drafted into leadership roles within the group. As a leader, one is expected to exemplify both mainstream society and the stigmatized group. The leader must help mainstream society feel comfortable and secure; but must also exhibit 'native performance' among the stigmatized group, to reassure them that although in frequent contact and association with the mainstream, he has not rejected them or begun to feel above them.[22] Deafened people who would otherwise be capable leaders often do not have sufficient capacity for native performance to reassure other deaf people that they are truly members of the group.

3.6 Finding a Refuge

What should you do when the 'Angel of Deaf' kisses your ear? After being rejected by the local deaf community, or perhaps being warned away from it by their doctor, audiologist, or counsellor, some deafened people look for support in hard-of-hearing groups, such as SHHH (Self-Help for Hard of Hearing People, Inc.). Many deafened people, while not feeling specifically rejected, do feel unsatisfied with the type of support they receive in both deaf and hard-of-hearing groups. The complaint is often that deaf people do not allow them to value both the Deaf culture and the Hearing culture, and that an all-or-nothing decision is expected. Yet at the same time, joining hard-of-hearing groups is no solution either. Many deafened people find that hard-of-hearing people cannot understand why amplification, loops, T-switches, and other assistive listening devices do not work for deafened people. In sum, neither deaf nor hard-of-hearing groups really understand the impact of the *change* from being hearing (or hard of hearing) to being deaf, and the resulting demands on the person, the family, and the work situation. At various times, in various places, deafened people have said, 'We need a group for people like us.'

In 1983, Jackie Metzger, Joe Weber, and John Shiels circulated a fifteen-page survey that yielded one hundred late-deafened responses and a workshop at ADARA (American Deafness and Rehabilitation Association). Regrettably, the national association of which they dreamed did not materialize at that time.[23]

In Britain, recognition of deafened adults can be traced back to 1923.[24] It is a sign of the age of such a group that one must lament the loss of its records, destroyed when the headquarters was bombed during the Second World War! The National Association of Deafened People (U.K.) was founded in 1984, but before the independent NADP was founded its members had been a segment of the British League for the Hard of Hearing and Deafened.[25]

Deafened social worker Michel David started a Deafened Adults Support Group at the Canadian Hearing Society head office in Toronto in 1986. This group was the seed of the Canadian Deafened Persons Association (founded 1990), which continues to meet. Many members also belong to the Association of Late-Deafened Adults (ALDA).

A support group for deafened adults that had been meeting at Ravenswood Hospital in Chicago suspended operations in the spring of 1986, leaving behind a craving for community. ALDA is considered to have been founded on 28 March 1987, on the occasion of a party for support group members and other late-deafened 'strangers.' Thirteen deafened people attended that party, hosted by Bill Graham. The association's name has been criticized for various reasons: 'late' also means 'tardy' and 'deceased,' and it is often sign-interpreted wrong (no, it isn't sign-interpreted NOT-YET DEAF). People think it refers only to people in late adulthood (i.e., old) or is limited to those who were already adults when they became deaf. Originally, ALDA defined its target membership as those who cannot hold regular conversations on an ordinary phone and feel in limbo among both deaf and hearing groups. Currently, the principle of self-identification governs: if you consider yourself deafened (or 'late-deafened'), you are. Some members became deaf during their preschool years, yet the combination of their early hearing memories and an education in the hearing culture makes them feel separate from other groups. The group includes those who are currently experiencing progressive hearing loss that is expected to continue to deafness.

By the way, the generally accepted way to sign 'deafened' is to point to the ears and then draw the A-hands down, wiggling at the wrists (HEAR-DETERIORATE).

Chapter 4

Professional Help

The first form of help deafened people usually encounter is professional help. Before they meet peers to avail themselves of peer help, and before they learn how to practise self-help, they consult with practitioners in a variety of professions. Professionals may be equipped with a fair background in dealing with hard-of-hearing people and/or the people who are called the Deaf Culture, and unsure which of this is applicable to a deafened client. If the client is your first and only deafened client, or you see only isolated cases, you will have little basis for evaluating how normal his problems and reactions are. Arguably the worst basis to use is how you think *you* would feel if you lost your hearing, because of the risk of transference. Unfortunately, this is also the most natural benchmark.

A number of books and journal articles have addressed acquired hearing loss; but these have focused little on what 'accepting deafness' means. Some contributions have been biographical and as such are insightful though not generalizable. Most other material reflects the medical model of deafness. Even more recent publications on late deafness[1] continue to focus on the physical/audiological rehabilitation or the vocational/occupational areas, and do not examine this condition from the perspective of psychosocial adjustment. Because of this, social workers may view adventitious deafness as only a sensory disability when it is also – and perhaps foremost – a social disability. Deafness shakes the foundations of one's identity and also isolates one from social interaction with family and friends. Only in the past ten years has this aspect of hearing loss come to the awareness of the social service community. When one medical researcher reported that 'many' clients had been in contact with a social worker (in contrast to 'few' having seen speech therapists[2]), we began to feel optimistic that social workers, counsellors, and human services professionals could help deafened people adjust. However, even deaf and deafened social workers have told us that they received negligible or no training in late deafness, even if they received some training in deafness.[3]

4.1 Traditional Intervention

4.1.1 Aural Rehabilitation

Aural rehabilitation, a service provided by audiologists, is perhaps the oldest and most common professional intervention provided for late deafness. Strictly speaking, aural rehabilitation has five components: (1) giving the individual a clear understanding of his hearing problem, (2) psychological adjustment for each patient (including the patient's family), (3) the fitting of a hearing aid when appropriate, (4) training in the use of residual hearing, and (5) speechreading.[4] Social workers must be aware when making a referral for aural rehabilitation that it may offer little or no counselling on the psychosocial aspects of late deafness.[5] We and other deafened people have observed that the assumptions behind the rehabilitation curriculum are driven by hard-of-hearing people, simply because they dominate most client rosters by their sheer prevalance in the population. Because they can apply their residual hearing to the exploitation of hearing aids, listening skills, and lipreading, hard-of-hearing people validate these strategies, proving that 'on average' they work for people with acquired *hearing loss*. As a result of this nondifferentiation, many clinicians have handed deafened people brochures and books by hard-of-hearing people, that essentially describe ways to cope successfully with *moderate to severe* hearing loss. As a result, the deafened person spends needless time wondering what is wrong with her.

On the bright side, 'adequate guessing' has been seen to be more important in lipreading than either residual hearing or length of time since becoming deaf.[6] In *normal* conversation, contextual evidence can contribute five to ten times as much information as sensory evidence.[7] Loss of hearing greatly reduces sensory evidence, limiting it to residual or amplified hearing and whatever can be lipread. Oral communication is more successful for good guessers, people with such phenomenal knowledge that they are familiar with many contexts, people moving in familiar circles, and people with the situational power to control their conversations.

> Researchers have observed, astutely, that the lipreader's visual focus on the speaker's lips can be disconcerting. I'll say. While my unwavering gaze convinced my high school teachers that I was an attentive scholar, many's the gentleman who thought I was trying to pick him up. Staring at people's lips is interpreted culturally.
>
> K.W.

The proponents of lipreading[8] argue that anyone can learn it (and that everyone probably should). Here, we respectfully submit our difference of opinion. Our highly personal observations support Thomas's remarks: 'While a few hearing impaired individuals are undeniably good lipreaders, the vast majority make little if any progress, even after prolonged attendance at lipreading class.'[9] However, because it provides visual cues, lipreading may determine whether or not a deafened person can make sense of vibro-tactile aids or hearing aids/cochlear implants. Note that even after lipreading the words successfully, the deaf or deafened person remains cut off from the intonations that mark the difference between straightforward and sarcastic comments, and token as opposed to enthusiastic praise, and other important nuances. We also find that even with good lipreading ability, we cannot reliably lipread the two-dimensional medium of television (despite this, much lipreading self-instructional material is on videotape).

Many of the strongest proponents of lipreading have some business interest in it; for our part, we do not teach sign language or have anything to gain by discouraging people from lipreading, or from adopting any alternative modes of communicating. In fact, we regularly use lipreading and work hard at it. People who cannot hear eventually *must* try to make some use of it. Lipreading is extremely difficult without residual hearing (something many people seem not to acknowledge). In the same way, trying to use residual hearing without lipreading is invariably harder than using the two combined. Our main concern is that deafened people should not place all their eggs in the one basket that represents the least change and effort for everyone else. Ironically, we find that the people we can lipread most easily are those who sign, whether or not they are actually signing at the time. This suggests to us – based on our sample of two – that the most critical quality is the sender's communication skill, not the receiver's lipreading skill. If deafened people's families would make the effort to change the way they communicate, it would likely help the deafened person to communicate in the old ways.

To assert that 'anyone' can learn to lipread is to mislead those people who for whatever reason just don't have the residual hearing or the cognitive capacity to do it effectively. It builds up their hopes that with just a little *more* effort, it will finally work. In the meantime ... stay home and bar the doors? The implication should never be made that failure so far has been due to inadequate effort on the deafened person's part. We think this is altogether too much pressure to put on someone who is already dealing with profound feelings of inadequacy, loss, and stigma.

4.1.2 Hearing Aids and Implants

Hearing aids pick up sound at a microphone, magnify it, and channel it directly into the ear canal, closer to the eardrum.

Every hearing aid can be tuned in a limited range of ways. Getting one isn't like buying a car – that is, the choice of make and model is not a 'consumer' choice. A qualified audiologist must be consulted to *prescribe* the right hearing aid that can be tuned to the optimal response.

Hearing aids may be of some benefit for a person with progressive hearing loss who is not yet completely deaf. Newer-style, digital hearing aids may be especially helpful for these people's adjustment. However, if too much of the speech range is inaudible regardless of loudness, amplification will not help the deafened person communicate. In sum, once a person is at the deafened stage, hearing aids are of little use, although they may provide some reassuring environmental awareness.

Cochlear implants and the brainstem implant are special varieties of 'hearing aids.' They have been intensively marketed to deafened adults who derive no benefit from amplification (conventional hearing aids). One often encounters materials which declare that implants are not hearing aids because the technology is completely different; although they are not amplifiers, we still think of them as hearing aids because they fill the same role in the social-communication sense. They consist of a portion surgically implanted in the user and an external sound processor. The sound processor is worn on the body like a personal stereo (newer models that are miniaturized for behind-the-ear wear have been developed). Sounds are picked up by a microphone and sent to the processor, which converts them into signals that are passed through the skin (by direct connection or wireless signal) to the implanted portion. Implants have become highly politicized and are a strong source of tension between the medical and Deaf communities.[10] Much of the tension revolves around the sensitive issue of paediatric implantation, which is of no relevance to the decision by a mature, informed adult to choose an implant. Another factor that caused friction in the deafened community was the original 'hard sell,' which was perceived as trading on the 'desperation and hopelessness' of deafness. On top of this, manufacturers involved networks of implantees to do their marketing for them.[11]

I never wanted a cochlear implant, but I have always respected the individual's right to make an informed decision to have one. I have always been happy to discuss CIs when I am not being assaulted by sales pitches and criticism for my position. A couple of the implantees on a cochlear implant panel I attended seemed to feel personally responsible for proselytizing for implants, even to the extent of being apologetic about the unsuccessful cases. I had to ask: 'How can we share information about CIs without the pressure and the sales pitch?' This sparked some interesting responses, and – I was glad to see – a bit of self-examination by the pro-implantation panellists. But immediately afterward, in the buffet line, another implantee accosted me and said, 'You made a very good point and I understand what you are saying, but I think you would be an excellent candidate for an implant. You should consider one.' You can make a person hear, it seems, but you can't make them listen.

K.W.

Uninformed people often believe that since a 'bionic ear' device now exists, it only makes sense that all deaf people should now rid themselves of their costly disability. It is understandable that people who have never been deaf would think so. However, social workers and counsellors need to know that not all deaf and deafened people are medically eligible for implants. Also, because of the complex nature of the devices, even those who are surgically acceptable may not be appropriate candidates. Implants do not repair the defect – they *bypass* it. The implant introduces electronic stimulation to the auditory nerves, which many people are able to learn to perceive as replacement for the sounds they once heard.

In a conversation I seem to have over and over, people who are considering implants (or sometimes their family members) approach me and ask, 'Are you happy with your implant?' I reply that I am as happy with my implant as I was before it. The implant is not capable of making me *happy.* It sometimes makes me function more easily, able to comprehend sound. I did not expect to become hearing, and I didn't. I had reasonable expectations, and I am not disappointed. I often leave it off. I would rather use a TTY than have difficult, guesswork telephone conversations. We use sign language around the house. I am never quite sure of the relevance of my happiness to anyone else, because our lives, circumstances, and values are likely quite different.

M.A.

Successful use of the implant depends on many factors, including the actual surgical outcome. Equally important is the implantee's capacity to learn to interpret the new auditory stimuli. Usually, the best implants do not deliver perfect blindfolded speech recognition. For 'good performance,' the user must be able to make sense out of context when about half the words are recognized. Also, because implantation is done on only one side, the sound perception provided gives no directional information; thus, the implant is likely to be less than satisfactory for those who are required to communicate in large groups or busy environments. Picking a message from a noisy background is not an easy task for electronics. Although the processor can be adjusted to make the best of the available situation, the result in multi-speaker environments may be ample perception of noise and talking, but difficulty understanding a specific speaker.

The implantee is free to swim and shower and play tennis, but the external processor that stimulates the electrode is an expensive electronic device that must be kept dry and safe. Undoubtedly, some people do sleep with the processor connected, but most remove it at bedtime. Occasionally, the processor malfunctions and must be repaired. While the processor is not connected, the user is as deaf as ever; hence, lipreading, signalling devices, and other coping and communication skills cannot be discarded.

My pure lipreading skills went from adequate to extremely poor soon after I received my cochlear implant. As my total dependence on lipreading decreased, so did the attention I paid to the skill. I can now lipread only when my processor is on. As a result, I find myself highly vulnerable when the batteries die (daily), when the wires need replacing (periodically), when I crack the case and damage the device through the activities of daily living, when I forget to pack it, and when I am in the locker room wrapped in a towel. Even when the implant is on, it is not a panacea. To my extended family and my business acquaintances, my implant is a magical solution to the tragedy of deafness. The ease of most of our direct conversations seems to prove that it has perfectly overcome my deafness. As a result, when we assemble in large groups for holiday parties or quarterly staff meetings, and my implant is of no benefit at all, they conclude that my disengagement must be caused by something else — perhaps disinterest, or self-absorption, or lack of intelligence. In fact, the utility of the implant varies widely, and in some cases it just sets me up for unreasonable expectations.

M.A.

Expectations are of the utmost importance. If they are too high, perfectly adequate performance can be disappointing. The implantee's expectations must be realistic, and so must those of significant others. Many candidates *describe* quite realistic expectations; and they hear the cautions in the candidate selection profile. However, realistic expectations can coexist with higher hopes. If the hopes are kept private in order to meet the selection criteria, and if the implant subsequently does not perform beyond reasonable levels, it will be difficult for the person (or their family and friends) to admit to and deal with the disappointment. In an assessment of expectations, consideration should be given to the nature and strength of any *secret hopes* as well as to those expectations people admit to.

At a cochlear implant information session, an audiologist was explaining various factors that affected speech recognition, and a minor factor noted was that sometimes 'full insertion' could not be achieved. (During surgery, as the tiny, coiled electrode array is threaded into the spiral passageway of the cochlea, the surgeon may encounter resistance or obstruction, and some of the electrodes may remain outside the cochlea, not in contact with the auditory nerve.) Regardless of the low incidence of partial insertion, or the fact that all of the electrodes are often not needed to get a good map, the audience – candidates, partners, and families – went into full-tilt rumination. Partial insertion was the unpredictable, uncontrollable factor that could foil their escape from deafness: the nameless fear now had a name. Since they attended the same clinic as one of us, we know they knew that performance varied and was subject to limitations. The attention they gave to this unlikely complication reveals just how much each of them was hoping to be the exceptional perfect outcome.

Candidates must understand clearly what the implant won't allow them to do with regard to physical activity, environmental exposure, medical procedures, and contacts with other electronic and magnetic devices. They must also understand the financial investment required to maintain the implant. Batteries, wires, holsters, add-on devices, insurance, aural rehabilitation, and 'remapping' all cost money. So does new processor technology, which will always come along and which will require further thousands of dollars of investment. Candidates should not be permitted to 'yeah yeah yeah' their way past these issues, no matter how eager they are to rid themselves of their deafness.

One of us has had an implant for almost ten years; the other has recently and reluctantly acquired one, for professional and economic reasons. We agree that implants, implantation surgery, and candidate selection have achieved impressive success rates (and we hope that no long-term side effects will appear, as happened with some breast enhancement prostheses). We know many implantees, and we have seen implants increase their confidence, and their control of speech quality.[12] On the other hand, we have also seen people say, 'I might as well have an implant because I have nothing left to lose.' This distresses us, because it indicates an emotional vulnerability that is not ideal ground for making the complex decision that major surgery entails.

Professionals should make sure the candidate is making an *emotionally* informed decision as well as a *medically* informed decision. The social worker or psychologist should help the candidate consider emotional questions, and should strive not to accept contrived 'right' answers of the kind that are oriented toward getting the candidacy approved. 'How will you feel if the implant is disappointing or ineffective?' 'How will you feel if deaf people criticize your choice to have the implant?' 'How do you expect to handle unrealistic expectations from your significant others?' The implant should not bear the entire responsibility for communication between the deafened person and significant others. We are encouraged if the deafened person sees the implant as a practical, perhaps economic, concession to employment and community functioning rather than as an answer to social isolation and emotional suffering. We are encouraged if the significant others have made equivalent efforts to meet the deafened person halfway, not just with moving their lips more slowly and clearly so that the deafened person can lipread, but (for instance) with gestures, notes, and fingerspelling (or home signs, if not going together to formal sign language classes).

Some implant teams have established careful screening techniques that address these issues. We hope that social workers are also aware of the adjustment issues and that they consider whether the candidate's consent is emotionally informed when making referrals to implant programs.

The difficulty of obtaining genuinely informed consent, either medically or emotionally, for this procedure is underestimated. People desire the implant because they are not very good communicators. Their great proficiency at giving the impression that they understand when they do not may be exceeded only by their desire to be accepted for implantation. Implant teams should anticipate misinformed consent and excessive expectations (particularly emotional expectations), and make exceptional efforts to deal with these through thorough counselling. The 'unidirectional, dutiful disclosure' involved in traditional consent is no longer enough; patient involvement has to be the new goal. It is a challenge to expand the idea of *consent* so that it becomes a process of informed patient participation in clinical decision-making, but it is necessary.[13] If patient involvement is ever relevant, it certainly is relevant in this situation, where not only the implant recipient but also her associates – both those aware of the implant and those who are unaware – will be conspicuously, continuously, and perpetually affected.

To develop the candidate's ability to honestly give emotionally informed consent, we advocate a reasonable moratorium period, rather than a rush to implant rapidly after onset of deafness. During the first few months or a year after becoming deaf, the person will not yet have reached emotional equilibrium, or explored her coping skills enough to answer questions about her own expectations and those of her significant others. This moratorium would do more than simply put the newly deafened person on a one-year waiting list; it would entail exposure to other deafened adults, both implanted and non-implanted. As appropriate, self-help training and relationship-centred follow-up would be provided before proceeding with implantation.

4.1.3 Vocational Rehabilitation

Vocational rehabilitation, or VR, is another common focus for counselling. Deafened people often believe – or are told – that they are no longer able or welcome to do their former jobs (or pursue the careers they were in the middle of preparing for), and sometimes this is true. Jobs in which the principal activity is the processing of auditory information (e.g., switchboard operator) are not amenable to deaf workers. We wouldn't want to close the door entirely on someone's choice of career, but we would prefer not to be flying through a deaf air traffic controller's airspace. More typically, people jump to the conclusion that their former work is no longer amenable simply because they can't do it the same *way* they always have. Many deafened people have retired early, demoted themselves, or discontinued their climb up the corporate ladder because they feel unable to function in meetings and on the telephone.

A well-informed VR counsellor can help a deafened person identify the various assistive devices and services (e.g., real-time transcription, interpreting) that will minimize career disruption. Where a change of job is inevitable, both counsellors and clients may be encouraged by the numbers of deafened people who have found new careers. Many others have continued to practise their old profession, such as counselling and teaching, but with deaf clients instead of the mainstream clients they formerly had, or expected when they trained for their profession.

4.1.4 Assistive Devices

Another topic often covered in VR counselling is the acquisition of assistive devices. Plenty of gadgets and gizmos have been created that aid daily living for deafened people. Among our favourites: television caption decoders (now incorporated into most television sets); TTYs (telephone keyboard attachments that permit typed conversations over telephone lines); modems that permit computers to function as TTYs (to obviate the stupid little keyboards most TTYs are made with); fax machines and e-mail; vibrating wake-up alarm clocks; and various flashing signal systems to indicate when the phone is ringing, the baby is crying, the door is being knocked on, or indeed the house is burning down. Two-way paging permits TTY and e-mail access on the road, and even offers fax and voice synthesis to leave text messages on voice-mail machines.

Counsellors help clients learn about these devices, and explain how to find them (most aren't sold at the local Radio Shack, unfortunately). For eligible clients, they also explain how to arrange government subsidies. Counsellors help the client learn how to use the devices, or find someone who will help him develop proficiency with them. One of us sat staring at a brand-new TTY for two days, working up the nerve to try making the first call, unsure whether the protocol described in the instruction manual would really be the way the world worked. (It was; it worked out fine.)

Our Favourite Technologies /
Vibrating alarm clocks
Flashing signals for door, baby, fire, smoke
Closed captions
Fax
TTY
TTY-modem
TTY-cell phone adapters
Alphanumeric vibrating pagers and paging services with
   TTY gateways
E-mail and WWW
Two-way paging to TTY, fax, voice message, e-mail

We love technology. The trouble with technical rehabilitation is that the uncomfortable client can stretch it out to be The Whole Issue. We know a number of deafened adults who have managed to entirely avoid emotional coping for years and years by focusing on technical acquisitions and VR issues.

4.2 Counselling

The most marked counselling requirement that emerged from interviews with deafened people was for family or relationship-centred counselling. With no exceptions, deafened people identified more problems with their relationships with significant others than with their own individual coping, and they recommended that deafened people receive professional counselling centred on those relationships. Almost none had been able to get this. Some had been turned down by programs that were unable to cope with their problem. Others merely received referrals for the types of professional help discussed in the previous section. The message: 'You need to learn to listen and get by with less hearing.'

Those who received individual-centred counselling received this secondary message: 'You had a loss, you need to grieve.' But conventional loss-grief counselling is missing the key element of identity adjustment. Being deafened is not like becoming hard of hearing, nor is it like always having been deaf, yet these are the only two conditions that most programs are equipped to handle. The material in the first three chapters will improve the effectiveness of individual-centred counselling. The following section describes the lessons learned from deafened adults about their counselling needs, including approaches to relationship-centred help.

4.3 Relationship-Centred Help

Many of the consequences of becoming deaf have a direct impact on the family. Clearly, deafness interferes with communication in any family that has depended on oral speech, and communication is a requirement for family relations. In the individual-centred model of professional help, these consequences are dealt with by advising the deafened person of the need for his family to adjust. Research has shown that this just isn't adequate. Deafened adults have identified the rehabilitation of family relationships as their greatest need – and as the greatest shortcoming of the services they received.[14] *Every effort must be made to involve the family in the counselling sessions*, even when the presenting problem was individual-centred. (The comments in this section that refer explicitly to the family will apply equally well to any similar group of significant others.)

For starters, the deafened person may still be feeling too inept, or embarrassed, or intimidated by the hearing loss to carry off the assurance required to convince his family to change and to help them know how to change. He may not even be sure what it will take to achieve fully functional communication, or what kind of emotional support he needs. Possibly more importantly, however, any fair negotiation requires that the parties have equality, and the deafened person in the family is *not* equal, and knows it. Acquired deafness is an acquired 'defect,' and this diminishes his power in negotiating with the family. Deafened women may face the additional deficit of unequal gender power.

This is where the social worker adds an important factor. The social worker can provide more than information and referrals; she can be an *advocate* for the deafened person. Within the safe, controlled environment of counselling, using a variety of techniques to create interactions of certain types, she can expose dysfunctional syndromes and patterns that risk harming family relationships. Having brought these things to light, she is also there to help resolve problems in a constructive way– and if blame is to be placed for letting the genie out of the bottle, then she is there to help the deafened person shoulder the burden. By initiating these discussions, the social worker can show the reasonableness of the needs of the deafened person and place them in the family context. This can validate the deafened person's tentative perceptions of what his needs are, while diminishing the family's objections to needs they perceive as peculiar, inconvenient, or excessive. Once problems are in the open, the social worker can help the deafened person and the family learn and practise equitable solutions.

Family dysfunctions are complex and sometimes carefully concealed. For social workers, complementary experience with family dysfunctions is a distinct asset. With experience, a social worker becomes familiar with even the better-hidden dysfunctions, and learns how to draw out the evidence and help the family to recognize it as well. At that point, the family can be guided toward a resolution. As we mentioned earlier, the trouble working with deafened people and their families is that most social workers – even deaf social workers and social workers who have studied deafness interventions specifically – have never studied adult onset deafness.The following section is for social workers without extensive experience with deafened clients, and discusses the dysfunctional syndromes that emerge among deafened adults.

4.3.1 Dysfunctional Family Responses

Various dysfunctional syndromes can occur. Sometimes they represent a conflict between the family and the deafened person's preferences; other times the deafened person is fully in agreement with the family, or in fact the initiator of the syndrome. It is always possible that the deafened person and/or the family will refuse to abandon these syndromes. Nevertheless, the social worker will want to explore any possible dysfunctions and help the family with difficult changes if they are open to it. We will discuss the following dysfunctional responses:

- Counterfactual thought
- Communication disruption
- Role disruption
- Unrealistic expectations
- Overprotectiveness
- Misplaced efforts
- Problem depreciation
- Abuse

4.3.1.1 Counterfactual Thought

As in any adverse situation, counterfactual thought can occur. We rarely seek explanations for good fortune, but it is common to see a negative situation in terms of the differences between reality and the normal or desirable situation. Explanations, whether they are accurate or not, rarely help reverse or reduce the adversity. Nor does it help much to identify causes. Deafened people spend plenty of time wondering why they were 'chosen' to become deaf, but eventually practicality forces them to redirect their thoughts toward coping. Families – who themselves still cope just fine – may need help to move on from such ruminations as, 'Did we cause it?' Perhaps this obsession with causes is a means to avoid the harder question: 'How do we cope with it?' The family needs to stop looking back with regret and start moving forward toward acceptance, because their ruminations will hinder the deafened person when she *is* ready to move on.

4.3.1.2 Communication Disruption

Often with hearing loss, the difficulty with communication means that no one tries to communicate unless there is a specific need to get a particular message across. There is no longer any communication that has no specific 'message,' yet it is this latter kind of communication that is vital for building rapport and communicating empathy, and for social learning.

Rapport is also fostered through a shared sense of humour. Either the deafened person or the family may be unable to see the humour in everyday situations arising from deafness. If either is unable to laugh about these, no bonding can occur through them, and overtures with humorous intent will fail. In the same vein, if the family sees humour but the deafened person does not, hurt may result. This commonly occurs when jokes are added to the family lexicon with their roots in some error of lipreading or hearing. Henry Kisor's book *'What's That Pig Outdoors'* was titled after his lipreading corruption of 'What's that big loud noise?' asked by a child who was curious about a particularly noteworthy episode of flatulence. His autobiographical premise was that remarking on his errors of comprehension did not bother him, and that sharing the amusement was a cornerstone of his success at growing up deaf. Many deafened people would like to say the same, but find it wearing to always be the unwitting source of humour, especially since they had once been able to understand without such mistakes.

On the other hand, if the deafened person sees humour but the family does not, the family will feel awkward and may avoid the topic, and the deafened person may perceive this as rejection. The family may fail to see the humour because they associate it with stigma and are not quite ready to accept the association with it; or the humour may be at the expense of hearing people, which makes them feel culpable. When significant others no longer share the same humour wavelength, communication is disrupted.

4.3.1.3 Role Disruption

When one member of the family is no longer able to communicate in the conventional way, the family sometimes responds by dividing up the communication-related tasks among other family members. The family structure changes as a result of this, and roles are altered. The family considers this to be simply a practical issue and sees nothing wrong with having the hearing partner do all the parenting, for example. When hearing children get into a habit of addressing the hearing father (let's say) out of convenience, and both parents acquiesce to this, the deafened mother's authority may be undermined. By the time she realizes she is playing a less significant role in the children's life and seeks to regain equal parenting status, too much damage may have been done. To avoid this problem, conscious efforts must be made to maintain equal parenting roles. The children need to be able to address both parents equally, and if this means learning sign language as well as spoken language, this should be considered.

Often the deafened person will continue to speak and the hearing partner (or another family member) will sign or gesture or write or mouth clearly, thus becoming the conduit of all communication with the deafened person. Soon enough, other family members and strangers begin to communicate through this pathway. The assistance and interpretation become so intensive and continuous that the hearing partner begins to anticipate the deafened person's needs, to respond on her behalf, and to develop strong views about what it is like to be deafened. The hearing partner loses awareness that he does not actually have first-hand experience, while the deafened person goes through life living everything as pre-digested by the hearing partner, learning about information and decisions after the fact. The hearing partner makes all the social arrangements and 'for efficiency' begins to act as a proxy or a surrogate in making plans and choices.

When the deafened person develops a dependence on this person as the provider of interpretation, she is vulnerable to the partner's reliability. Sometimes the partner is not there, or chooses when and how much information to convey. The deafened person will eventually experience a situation where she feels left out and lacking alternatives, because she has not developed the ability to function independently. Relying on interpreting is not dependence, because there are many sources of interpreting. Relying on one *particular* interpreter *is* dependence, as there is no alternative access when that person is unavailable to objectively interpret.

Role disruption can also be caused by dysfunctional adjustment of the deafened person. When he is too absorbed in his own misery, he can't fulfil the role of helper to his partner, who has her own day-to-day problems to deal with: 'You're not there for me any more.' The hearing partner needs a shoulder to cry on: all her other problems don't go away when her husband becomes deaf. If he is wrapped up in his adjustment struggles, he becomes emotionally unavailable to her.

4.3.1.4 Unrealistic Expectations

The family will often not let the deafened person 'give in,' as it characterizes acceptance of the deaf condition. The focus is on 'overcoming' deafness. The optimists insist that deafness or at least its difficulties will go away over time: either hearing will return or lipreading will become perfectly effective. The operative fallacy here is that if *any* person with *any* degree of hearing loss *ever* managed with oral communication and lipreading, *our* deafened person can do it. While this is couched as a vote of confidence in the resourcefulness, resilience, and superiority of *our* deafened person, the real benefit is to the partner, family, and friends, who will not need to change. The core expectation is that it is possible for the old communication modes to succeed. People may need to shout or speak slowly, but there is no need to consider home signs or ASL.

In the family counselling context, the therapist needs to be attuned to 'groupthink.' In groupthink, a group adopts certain tenets and rejects contrary positions as 'enemy' views.[15] Incon-sistent observations are ignored or discounted, and members self-censor to ensure that threats to the cherished positions are excluded. There may be conflict not only between the deafened person and family members, but also between those family members who have decided to accept change and those who are defending the group norm.

Sometimes a family will urge the deafened person not to ask for help – to strive for super-independence. Like the premise that deaf children who learn sign language will be too lazy to learn English, a deafened person who asks for help in this world of auditory tasks may be seen not as giving in on one thing, but rather as giving up on everything and anything. A deafened person who expects never to need any functional help will soon find herself overcompensating, which can easily lead to frustration over inevitable failures. A key personal gain in the process of adjusting to deafness is finding in oneself the willingness to go to a hearing person at an information counter and ask that a phone call be made. The alternative is hours and hours of frustration and anger over the lack of public TTYs (which, while a worthy cause of protest, is not a fast way to get a ride home when the car breaks down). This is not merely a stiff-upper-lip, bootstraps issue. In 1989,[16] the Deaf Culture adopted the rallying cry, 'Deaf people can do anything except hear.' Families and deafened people need to 'hear' the last two words of that slogan as clearly as the first five. Many of the barriers that deaf people experience are caused by the environment and its inaccessibility by means other than hearing. No amount of willpower is going to make a pay phone without a TTY work for a deaf person.

4.3.1.5 Overprotectiveness
Overprotectiveness can be the result of the unreasonable expectations discussed in the previous item: 'You should not let people know you are deaf. They will look down on you. I am only protecting you from hurt.'

Some families try to protect the deafened person from disappointment by encouraging him to 'be realistic' about goals.

Translation: 'Don't entertain the same set of expectations you previously had.' The apparent motive is to protect him from disappointment. The problem with this attitude is that it is based on the assumption – at least partially shared – that he is less capable than before. Many deafened people have been counselled to take practical rather than academic training, and to focus on job security rather than career rewards.[17] It is always someone else's probable discrimination that these advisers _(family or counsellors) are thinking of, never their own. The deafened person's indignation over diminished career prospects can be countered by ascribing to him delusions or a personality disorder. Deafened people are often advised to expect less and not rock the boat. If the lesser career can be satisfying, this can be reasonable, but for many deafened people it is a recipe for deferred frustration.

Some family members will focus on the deafened person as a model of sainthood, inspiration, and all-round infallability for having gone through the ordeal of deafness. Whether conscious or unconscious, this is plain condescension. It reduces the deafened person to a single experience, and suggests that she is held to lesser expectations, that she need do nothing else but survive the trauma to be considered a model of achievement. Professing admiration precludes complaints of patronizing treatment: How can we patronize someone we explicitly look up to? Normal relations can only occur when family members perceive one another through a normal lens. Putting any member of the family on a pedestal for any reason denies that person the right to a normal amount of human weakness, fears, and failings. The idolized family member must either be saintly, or conceal her true self. Either of these only serves to constrain her equal membership in the family.

4.3.1.6 Misplaced Efforts
Many families are eager to help but inclined to 'cherry picking,' where the family members pick and choose how they would prefer to help, whether or not they have identified the most needed or wanted types of help. The deafened person is

expected to be grateful, and if he is not, the family resents the lack of appreciation.

Help is equally confounded when the family expects the deafened person to know what help is needed – to provide a 'shopping list' of help requirements. The deafened person has almost as little experience with deafness as the other family members and often can't judge how useful a certain kind of help is until after he has experienced it. Consistency cannot be expected. The value of a certain type of help can change from day to day as the adjustment to deafness changes.

Automatic empathy for the deafened person's loss – loss of access and loss of abilities – is misplaced. This is no different from pity. The deafened person needs the family to empathize with his difficulties and aspirations, as he perceives them, at each step of the adjustment process. After he has absorbed the loss initially, he is more likely to need empathy with his hopes and support for his retained abilities and new possibilities. He needs them to empathize with the need for change, and he needs help in making change constructive and easy and free of blame and regret – even though this isn't easy, as there will constantly be doubts and regrets.

4.3.1.7 Problem Depreciation

Many deafened people report that their families and friends diminish their difficulty. The crisis is belittled: 'Get over it,' 'You think you're the only person with problems.'

Families depreciate the crisis by suggesting that they are suffering equally. The process is all about their own pain: 'You don't realize how hard it is to talk to you.' These family members own a share of the *suffering* but see the *problem* as belonging entirely to the deafened person. Problem depreciation seems to be a matter of misplaced centre.

In these families, deafness is not the family's problem: 'You're the one who can't hear – we can hear you just fine.' Rather, it is a *medical* problem. The family expresses willingness to support the deafened person in *her* challenge to deal with *her* problem, but fundamentally refuses to see it as a *family* problem. To put this in perspective, one person who became deafened simultaneously to acquiring other disabilities described her family's unlimited and painstaking help with her toileting needs in stark contrast to their refusal to talk about her deafness.[18] A social worker's intervention may help that family see that their inability to communicate *to* the deafened person is just as much of a problem as the deafened person's ability to hear them.

In the early stages of adjustment, the family (just like the deafened person) may refuse to make any permanent adaptations to deafness because they are convinced that it is only a matter of time before this case is 'cured' – before the loss is reversed and everything goes back to normal. In the first place, the physician and audiologists should have disabused the family of these notions.[19] If this kind of resistance is apparent to the social worker, the family may need more discussion directed at creating more reasonable expectations and more active adjustment and support for the deafened person.

4.3.1.8 Abuse

Abusers will seize on any excuse and opportunity. Deafness probably does not turn one's partner into an abuser where there was no potential abuser, but some deafened people have found themselves feeling trapped in a family or relationship with a partner who turns to abuse. The abuser seizes on deafness as a source of disappointment and justification for punishment.

The situation is even worse if the deafened person feels the partner may be right, and accepts the blame and abuse. The deafened person tolerates the abuse out of fear that deafness has destroyed any value or appeal they might have had to other potential partners. Out of fear of loneliness, they excuse the abuse, so that the abuser doesn't even have to try to be a good partner. Deafened people who have left an abusive relationship are better off and soon realize the groundlessness of their earlier fears; many of them do find other mates, usually far more empathetic to their deafness. Hearing people and men do not hold any monopoly on being abusive mates; some abusers are deaf, and some are women.

Dysfunction Summary: Danger Signs

The social worker should observe for each of these potential patterns using both passive and active methods. The former involve observation, and asking for opinions, feelings, and reports; the latter involve creating interactive situations in the counselling session that will bring out these signs.

Dysfunction may exist if the counsellor observes or the deafened person reports that:
- The family ruminates on why the deafness occurred.
- Communication is described in terms of transfer of messages rather than rapport.
- The family seems uncomfortable talking about deafness with humour.
- The deafened person's mistakes are described as endearing standing jokes.
- One or more hearing members have assumed certain roles that the deafened person now performs less, especially parenting or relationships with adult parents.
- Significant others interpret for the deafened person (this often can be observed in a clinic), or worse, they answer on the deafened person's behalf.
- The partner feels that the deafened person is not emotionally available to support other crises and problems.
- The family uses terms such as 'giving in' to the deafness negatively and 'overcoming' deafness positively.
- The family thinks the deafened person is unrealistic or needs to be reasonable about expectations.
- The family thinks that notwithstanding other deaf and deafened people's experiences, *their* deafened person doesn't need us to sign, gesture, or write.
- There are disagreements among the hearing members of the family regarding what they owe the deafened person in the form of support.
- The family is concerned about the deafened person being dependent.
- The family is concerned about other people stigmatizing the deafened person.

- The family wants to protect the deafened person from other people's attitudes and actions.
- The family describes the deafened person in 'saintly' terms: 'inspiration' and so on.
- The family feels that the deafened person does not ask specifically enough for help or is inconsistent in what help she wants and when she wants and doesn't want it.
- The family uses terms such as 'get over it' or suggests that everyone has problems.
- The family identifies their own suffering as equal to or greater than the deafened person's.
- The family insists that it is a medical problem or a problem internal to the deafened person and refuses to see a shared problem.
- There are signs of abuse. This can mean physical and emotional abuse of the deafened person, or abuse of alcohol, or a chemical dependency.
- The deafened person exhibits enabling behaviours regarding abusive behaviour.
- The deafened person believes he would not find another partner if the present partner left him.

4.3.2 Clinical Interventions

4.3.2.1 Categories of Interventions
Interventions can be made on several levels with different clients.

At the **individual** level, the counsellor can offer *post-trauma* counselling interventions, such as bereavement/loss counselling and *identity transformation/transition* counselling (see Chapter 2). The social worker can also offer training interventions – for example, *communication reconstruction* and *environmental adaptation* (aids for daily living). The social worker should also conduct appropriate outcome evaluations to ensure that the communication is successful (see Section 4.3.2.3) and that the client is using the aids comfortably and effectively.

The social worker can also help the client find healthy *outlets and pastimes*. We hope it is clear by now that handing the client a

slip of paper with the address of the deaf club will not be sufficient to propel the client to follow through and achieve a healthy
lifestyle. While it is important for the deaf person to exercise
self-determination and take responsibility for herself, we also
suggest that the social worker exert some pressure on her to
counteract the internal forces working against social competence. We recommend deafened self-help groups as a pathway
to healthy outlets and pastimes; unfortunately, these are too
often not available. A social worker acquainted with a number
of deafened clients might facilitate the creation of a deafened
self-help group. Part II of this book describes the structure, function, and operation of self-help groups; also, we describe them
for the professional in Section 4.6.

At the **family** level, the social worker can help with *bereave-
ment/loss* issues and help the family work through what has happened: help them understand the process their deafened family
member is entering, and help them deal with their own sense of
loss. Functionally, the family may need help to *comprehend* the
changes to expect, particularly with progressive hearing loss,
and may need guidance in *reconstructing communication*. Group
counselling sessions are often useful for making both emotional
and practical adjustments.

4.3.2.2 Specifics and Starting Points

Most of the dysfunctions, once identified, can readily be
addressed with professional social work interventions: individual counselling, group counselling, skills training and evaluation. Individual exercises, behavioural contracts, and psychotherapy can be used.

The clinical social worker can make use of Table 4.1 as a point
of departure in devising customized interventions for client
families. Note that being 'in' a stage is not the same thing as
being 'stuck' in a stage. How fast a client transits through a
given stage depends on individual factors. Unless the client or
the client's family or colleagues identify that something is a
problem, dysfunctional family responses or evidence as indicated below must be seen.

TABLE 4.1
Adjustment problems and potential clinical interventions

Stage	Example of evidence of a problem	Example exercises
Identity confusion	Problems at work, problems in the family, feeling unsatisfied or dysfunctional; can't communicate effectively; talking too much, comprehension mistakes; friction over perceived inattentiveness. This might more usually be noticed as a problem apparent to the therapist in clients who have pre-presented for a different, or merely general, family dysfunction	Referral to clinical audiology; client(s) to return for follow-up after audiology; assist client to comprehend meaning of diagnosis, acknowledge permanence, also express any fears, e.g., of further 'betrayals,' e.g., 'what if I lose my vision?'
Identity comparison	Loss of hearing as a source of pleasure	Individual exercise: explore non-aural pleasure, pre-existing and new sources of visual entertainment and self-expression
	Dependent on partner to communicate with others	Behavioural contract: the partner withdraws the extensive support 'services' and the deafened partner tries going to some functions alone or with supports provided in the community, e.g., real-time captioning
	Neglecting personal relationships; relationship becoming only about the deafness	Behavioural contract: the deafened person to do something the partner enjoys; think of 5 ways to make that activity more enjoyable for self
	Embarrassment of being deaf	Individual-centred exercise to renormalize: therapist arranges to introduce the client and significant others to a 'custom-selected' reference group, deaf people who possess attributes the client considers admirable, e.g., intelligence, professional achievement, athletic ability

TABLE 4.1 (*continued*)
Adjustment problems and potential clinical interventions

Stage	Example of evidence of a problem	Example exercises
	Perception that deafness is the worst thing that could happen	Individual exercise: deafened person to do volunteer work with others in need; create potential to compare deafness with other experiences that are truly worse, but also to create opportunities for positive feedback about functionallty
	Description of problem is entirely external, e.g., anger about discrimination, job loss	Deal with presenting problem at face value, e.g., income maintenance, but use the clinical contact to explore impact of deafness in other areas of life
Identity concession	Spouse is tired of time the deaf partner spends pursuing support group activities	Behavioural contract: deafened person to try a reduced level of support group attendance and new activities to do with partner Substitute therapy: family/couple to participate in family-centred self-help sessions (using support group rules)
	Support group doesn't satisfy the perceived need	Psychotherapy to determine reason (may not be possible to solve behaviourally)
	Support group validates work dysfunctions, but the client cannot act on the recognized need for changes	Determine if there is any legal violation (e.g., reasonable accommodation regulations); if so, refer to formalized channels Work group education/counselling/mediation Psychotherapy about problems with confrontation and conflict
Activism	Work problems, e.g., discipline, not completing work; family problems, e.g., marriage in jeopardy; general social isolation: regretted loss of dear friends over deafness; individual dysfunction, e.g., observation of obsessive/compulsive behaviours, self-perceived as over-committed to activism	Behavioural contract: 'let it go,' act on only (for example) one issue per week Psychotherapy: diagnose whether condition arises from clinical OCD/OCPD and treat accordingly

TABLE 4.1 (*concluded*)
Adjustment problems and potential clinical interventions

Stage	Example of evidence of a problem	Example exercises
Depression	Chronic withdrawal from social interaction; cessation of favourite non-aural pastimes (e.g., attending baseball games, sewing/cooking); noticeable changes of appetite; excessive procrastination; repetitive self-derogations and expressing feelings of worthlessness; devaluing personal possessions	Usual treatments, e.g., exercise, diet, medical
Individual exercise: seek substitute activities if old sources of pleasure are no longer satisfactory; try resuming activities that were curtailed when deafness was first confronted
Psychotherapy to deal with or anticipate depression (in ongoing client, might be considered pre-emptively as stage of activism peaks)
Individual exercise: document the achievements made through activism, e.g., biographical essay, *curriculum vitae*, web page, journaling, etc.

4.3.2.3 Outcome Evaluation for Communication Improvement Interventions

While communication dysfunction is familiar to social workers, the situation of deafened adults and their families may present it in an unfamiliar form. The communication breakdown is not merely a conflict of understanding; it lies in the very mechanics of communication. The novelty arises from the fact that communication serves two purposes: *transmitting content* and *establishing and maintaining relationships.* In the next section, various options for communication are discussed, from sign language to transcription. The social worker will seek a solution that best meets the needs and values of the people involved.

For outcome evaluation, the social worker needs to incorporate both facets of communication in any measures: the *message* needs to get through, and the deafened person needs to perceive appropriate *relationship* value, of which *inclusion, affection, respect* and *autonomy* are the most important. The hearing members of the family also need to perceive that they are autonomous and

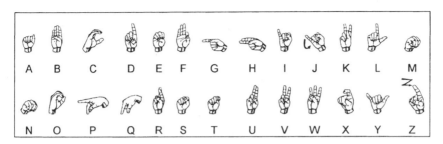

Figure 4.1: North American one-handed fingerspelling alphabet

respected. 'Communication' that achieves only the message or the relationship facet needs further development.

4.4 Sign Language and Interpreting

4.4.1 Gestures, Fingerspelling, and Home Signs

The most basic form of manual communication is simply *gesturing*. Almost everyone gestures a little, and many gestures are universally understood. There is nothing peculiar about gesturing.

When gestural communication becomes systematized and is used for a larger share of total communication, it can be called *home signs*. For instance, the home sign for 'eat' may look like one hand spooning food from the plate (the other hand) to the mouth. This is not the American Sign Language sign for EAT, but in a family when someone is trying to get the concept of mealtime through to the deafened person, it will do the job. Over time, many families develop robust vocabularies of original signs that everyone in the family understands. These go a long way toward equalizing communication so that everyone participates.

Many deafened people and their families learn the fingerspelling alphabet (Figure 4.1). *Fingerspelling* allows people to sign words by spelling them one letter at a time. This isn't sign language, any more than penmanship is English composition, but it is a fundamental tool. Sign language signs represent concepts (as English words do). Fingerspelling is used in sign language for proper names and technical terms and other bits of detail. However, fingerspelling can help the deafened person improve communication with deaf people. By fingerspelling the

English word in context, the deafened person can ask the deaf person to show the corresponding sign. This way, a vocabulary of signs can be built.

Deaf people can fingerspell very quickly. Many deafened people with a lot of signing experience struggle to read fingerspelling at the speed that deaf people and interpreters usually produce it. Deafened people do not need to hold themselves up to this standard in order to benefit. Fingerspelling is a big convenience when lipreading falters and there is no paper handy, and we really appreciate it when we are across a crowded room, on opposite sides of a plate glass window, or in two cars side by side at a stop light!

> Kids love fingerspelling, the same way they love all secret codes. Our daughter has been fingerspelling individual letters since before she was two. At the same age she could fingerspell the words B-U-S and B-E-E (which tend to be spelled as such in sign language). At age three, when we couldn't lipread a word she couldn't sign, she told us she had an 'I-D' (idea). Her preschool classmates can all spell all the letters too. In the right family environment, children will happily help communicate with sign language.

4.4.2 'Englishy Sign'

Learning to sign will not make a deafened person lose his residual hearing or his skills in speaking, writing, or lipreading English. Nor will using sign language prevent his hearing children from learning and using English. These absurd suggestions are propagated as scare tactics by those who oppose sign language. Many deafened adults talking to hearing people through an interpreter will voice for themselves, using sign language for receptive communication only. The absence of feedback, of hearing one's own voice, can cause speech to deteriorate, but learning to sign will have no effect at all, especially if speech is used just as much as before. How can learning to sign interfere with an adult's ability to write in English? How can signing with parents stop a hearing child from speaking English? Consider that that child is bombarded with television stimuli and surrounded by other relatives who hear, and by hearing classmates. The only plausible impact of learning to sign is that it will decrease the deafened person's motivation to persist with more effortful forms of communication, specifically lipreading.

Most deafened adults who take up signing start out using much the same grammatical structure as they would when speaking English, and they often speak and sign simultaneously. Since American Sign Language (ASL) and English have distinctly different grammars, it is not possible to speak one while signing the other without sounding incoherent in at least one version. For the deafened person, the English grammar tends to dominate, as it appears to do also for deaf and hearing people attempting 'simultaneous communication.'

> I learned sign language by mingling with people at the deaf club. I found it surprisingly easy to learn. For eight years I had been getting audible information visually, albeit with a great deal of effort. Even though their sign language was unfamiliar, these people were putting out the information visually in the first place. In fact, in four visits I had acquired a lot of vocabulary and was expressing entire thoughts in sign language. I had a bit of linguistic shock when I first encountered ALDA. Many of those people did sign, but they couldn't understand me until I stopped signing ASL and started to use the signs in English word order.
>
> M.A.

English also tends to dominate because many deafened people acquire a lot of their sign vocabulary from picture books of signs. It is impossible to learn any language simply by reading a dictionary, and it is much better to learn signs in person than from books. The diagrams of sign movements do not always convey what the sign looks like in reality. Although English-speaking

North America generally uses the same sign language, there *are* regional variations,[20] more in vocabulary than in grammar. Attending a sign language class is a way to find out how people in the local community produce a certain sign, which is more important than knowing how it is produced in Washington, D.C. (unless that is where you live). New learners, already frustrated that sign language is not universal, often complain that there 'shouldn't be' this variation. There is no point criticizing: English speakers in various parts of the continent may call the same sandwich a sub, a hoagie, a hero, or a 'big sandwich.' Synonyms, homonyms, and heteronyms exist in every language, and the student needs to accept that the same applies to sign language. Collections of sign pictures make it too easy to use the same sign for a given English word, regardless of meaning. Most books place little emphasis on the different signs available for different meanings – for example, 'pupil' (eye) versus 'pupil' (student).[21]

The importance of learning *ASL* grammar depends entirely on the deafened person's needs. To communicate with hearing family members, to use interpreters as a sole client, and to communicate with deaf people, counsellors, and even with many deaf people, the deafened person can achieve what she wants through Englishy signs.

Sign systems based on exact English do not warrant much mention here. Their purpose and merit, to the extent they have any, is to teach English to deaf children. Deafened adults already know English, so they have no need to learn the arcane mixture of suffixes, initializations, verb conjugations, and other devices that make these systems so burdensome for the visual-cognitive processing system.

4.4.3 *American Sign Language*

Notwithstanding the effectiveness of Englishy signing for many purposes, there is no particular eloquence to it. It is now widely acknowledged that ASL is a genuine language with rules of proper usage. Deafened people who are beginning to explore Deaf Culture and who have admired the skills of fluent users of sign languages may want to learn proper ASL.

If it is preferable to learn individual signs in person rather than from books, it is *essential* if one wants to learn the grammar of ASL. Most books skim over sign language grammar, perhaps mentioning that it is different. It is difficult to illustrate sentence structure in an accessible book.

We have experience with two approaches: sign language class and the deaf club. Sign language classes should be taught with the 'no voice' rule, which means starting with nothing but pantomime. The main complaint we hear about sign language classes is that strict teachers will not write a vocabulary word on the blackboard, insisting that there is no sign-to-word correspondence. They prefer to mime an explanation and build comprehension the same way children learn language. The frustrations of this may be greater for people recently deafened. Those with longer experience of deafness may be more accustomed to not immediately understanding things and figuring them out from context. Whatever it lacks in immediate gratification, the natural approach makes up for in learning by osmosis. Signed explanation rather than written English translation provides more models for how to use signs and gestures to communicate, and this is an advantage for the deafened person who wants to sign.

While both hearing and deaf teachers may be qualified and certified and equally professional, we prefer a deaf teacher for deafened people learning to sign. Even with 'no voice,' hearing teachers may unconsciously give an advantage to the hearing students because they can overhear the students muttering. Also, a deaf teacher can provide a role model and social entrée to a deafened person in a way that a hearing teacher cannot.

As a place to learn language, the deaf club functions in a unique way. Sign language teachers always encourage students to go to the deaf club, but the deaf club members are usually not eager to talk to poor signers. After all, they are at the deaf club for a respite from the frustration of working among hearing people, not to give free sign language lessons. Also, deaf club members may work around a newcomer's poor signing rather than giving feedback and correction, the same way English speakers tolerate broken English from foreigners. For a deafened person, the club is probably more worthwhile for the signing he sees used among others than for conversations he has directly.

With persistence, the newcomer may find someone willing to help him along, fill in vocabulary gaps, and explain what is going on. Kindly strangers are not always entirely well meaning. There are some common initiation pranks that can be distressing to deafened people, such as teaching the newcomer a name-sign for himself that is actually a part of anatomy or a bodily function, or teaching wrong signs (usually profanity) in place of proper signs for common phrases such as 'good morning' or 'May I please have a beer?' Forewarned is forearmed. Even though it is the club members themselves who are resisting the newcomer with bad signing, giving up on the club can be seen as a sign of 'bad attitude,' which will not help in future social forays.

Learning at least passable ASL will open doors to meeting deaf people for social, professional, and community interaction, and provide new access to a fascinating art medium – ASL poetry and theatre. The pursuit of ASL can be a long process, but most deaf people can adapt their signing to the person with whom they are talking, and will refrain from the most extreme idiomatic forms of ASL if they sense that the other person is doing their best just to sign basic ASL. Linguists refer to this as 'contact signing'[22] (referring to the improvisation of communication upon the contact between users of the two languages). (An older term is 'pidgin signed English' – PSE – although this is linguistically an inaccurate term.)

4.4.4 What Deafened People Need to Know about Interpreting

The most important thing deafened people may not know about interpreting is that the interpreter is responsible for communication. Except in situations where the interpreter is working for an audience, the interpreter is signing to meet the information needs of the specific deaf client. It is entirely legitimate for the deafened person to request an interpreter even if he only knows a little sign language. The client can watch the lips for lipreading purposes and the signs for building up a sign vocabulary. When the deafened person or the business calls the interpreting agency to request an interpreter, the request should specify someone who can sign Englishy and mouth clearly. Even if the specific request has not been made, a good interpreter will check before the assignment begins, and at suitable intervals, to make sure the client is satisfied.

Aside from the sign language lesson complete with vocabulary customized to your business or social needs, this is a big improvement over trying to lipread the other participants. The interpreter is not sitting in a random sequence of seats for the duration of the meeting, the way the speakers are. The interpreter sits in one spot, and you always know where to look to find the moving lips. Also, the interpreter is clearly there for a reason, so the other people present recognize that the individual is deaf and no awkward disclosure is needed. While this discloses the stigma, it also declares that the individual is doing something to get around the communication barrier instead of withdrawing, or expecting other people to speak in a stilted manner and continuously repeat themselves. It says, 'I don't view my condition as something to hide, so I do not expect you to think less of me.' Self-confidence counteracts other weaknesses.

The most difficult thing for a deafened person at first may be not knowing where to find interpreters. Most interpreters work through agencies either on a staff basis or freelance. Some larger businesses have established contacts with interpreting agencies in order to satisfy their obligations under the Americans with Disabilities Act or Rehabilitation Act (in the United States) or human rights laws (in Canada); so if the need is for corporate training, or a university class, or a conference, the human resources department or special needs department, or a convention planning firm can usually handle all the arrangements. A small business is more likely to be stumped, and it is useful to be able to guide them to possible resources. If no local sign language interpreting businesses are listed in the Yellow Pages or on the Internet, we suggest asking for a referral from an independent living centre or a hearing society. If these do not have an interpreting department that can make a booking directly, they will likely know how to find an interpreter. A website such as the Interpreters Network[23] can be a resource.

The deafened person will notice that some interpreters are easier to understand than others. That is normal. Some interpreters have better interpreting skills in some topic areas than others. Also, there are variations in signing and mouthing styles. If the deafened person finds that some interpreters are great and others are hard to follow, the booking agency should be told – in fact, it will appreciate this kind of feedback. You are not making a personal criticism when you ask that a certain interpreter not be assigned to you. It *is* helpful to try to figure out what it is about different interpreters that makes some easy to follow and others not. Sometimes the harder-to-understand interpreters can change the way they sign.

After a certain amount of working with the local pool of interpreters, I developed an A list (two people), a B list (a dozen or so), a C list (almost everyone else), and a Z list (two names: one who signed exact English and would *not* leave off that annoying grammatical flotsam and jetsam, and another who had a horrible hairdo that interfered with my visual attention). It was terrific once I let the agency know whom I preferred to work with and whom I preferred to avoid. It was interesting that the interpreters on my A and B lists were the same ones most deaf people preferred; in other words, there was nothing peculiar about my preferences just because English was my first language and I came to ASL late.

K.W.

4.4.5 What Interpreters Should Know about Deafened People

Unless she asks, the interpreter may not realize that a client is deafened and not just visiting or new to the community. If an unfamiliar client has 'normal' speech and indicates that he wishes to voice for himself, the interpreter should investigate whether the client is deafened. Interpreters tend to sign in the same type of sign language that the client expresses, and could end up signing a more fatiguing form of sign language that the deafened client doesn't really prefer. English requires more movements to express the same propositions, so this form of signing is more fatiguing and potentially more injurious to interpreters than regular ASL.[24] The only solution is for the interpreter to find out whether the client is deafened and then make a point of asking, or even testing, the client to see if ASL structure is more acceptable.

Interpreter Checklist
- Is the client voicing for himself? If a deafened client signs, it will probably be English-like, so try to voice his choices of English expressions.
- Don't assume that the client's expressive sign indicates receptive preference. Less strictly English signing, and even some ASL features, may be easier to follow.
- Ascertain whether the client prefers clear mouthing and generic signs (to avoid excessive fingerspelling).
- Modify the signs a little if this is required to keep the hands from blocking the client's view of the mouth.
- Get feedback from the client both by asking and by testing responses. Clients may be reluctant to criticize.

The interpreter should check how the deafened person feels about fingerspelling. For deaf people with good vocabularies or working in technical fields, the obvious solution is for the interpreter to fingerspell precise terms. In the case of deafened people, fingerspelling may be the worst thing to do. Our solution has been to combine the signs for the generic concept with mouthing of the exact word, because we can lipread well in context.

Deafened people often lack the assertiveness and directness

that deaf clients will exhibit in giving feedback to the interpreter. Deaf culture is much more direct than hearing culture, and this helps deaf clients express their preferences in ways that the interpreter can implement. Deafened clients often retain hearing culture norms. Sometimes we haven't mentally adjusted to viewing the interpreter as a service professional (rather than a social acquaintance), and we maintain the 'polite fictions,' saying that things are 'fine, fine,' to spare the acquaintance's feelings. We may feel insecure about giving feedback that signs appeared to be wrong because often the interpreter has been signing years longer than we have. We are also vulnerable to the 'anything is better than nothing' philosophy, so that our gratitude for being able to participate at all outweighs our expectation of easy participation.

> I felt awkward sitting in union contract negotiations watching the interpreter repeatedly signing 'drug plan' (the employee benefit) as though it referred to illicit drugs rather than prescribed medications. (There are different signs.) The peculiar image of illicit drugs being planned as an employee benefit made my mind wander; mentally, I had to make the transition and substitute the proper concept each time it came up because I felt uncomfortable saying anything that would make the interpreter feel bad.
>
> K.W.

4.5 Real-Time Transcription

Deaf people growing up with sign language have access to the hearing world through sign language interpreters. Even if they later go on to become fluent in sign language and eventually to prefer using interpreters, deafened people – with very few exceptions – begin the deaf portion of their lives as non-signing people. In fact, many cannot lipread. We often can still speak. Except where vision or cognitive skill is also lost, we still have all our former ability to read English. Regardless of whether we eventually learn sign language, transcription into text is an essential form of interpreting for every deafened person, at least temporarily.

It seems that public assembly and broadcast applications (i.e., television captioning) have been quicker to adopt real-time transcription. A great, hidden need relates to one-to-one interpreting situations, to allow deafened people to fully understand doctor appointments, parent/teacher meetings, and legal dealings; and to allow them to participate in the same fast-paced, complicated business dealings they carried on before deafness. A doctor cannot obtain 'informed consent' for surgery if she hasn't gotten the full story through to the deafened patient, even if she is confident that the patient somehow correctly understood the questions and provided an accurate and comprehensive medical history. What could be more appropriate than transcription at the hospital bedside of a newly deafened person? In this situation, the deafened patient is full of questions yet bereft of any means to communicate with a medical staff that is too busy to handwrite all the things they would simply *say* to a hearing patient. Clearly, a deafened person needs transcription just as much as a born-deaf person needs an interpreter at his or her doctor's office appointment. And we can't attain our professional potential by relying on the half of the story we get from lipreading or notes. Access means the ability to attain our potential, regardless of our deafness. Many access laws back up this right, but implementation sometimes lags behind. Thus, the deafened person has to cope not only with his own adjustment, but also with the too-common shortage of community resources. Real-time transcription is the key to access.

When a late-deafened support group was first formed in Chicago, communication was facilitated by a typewriter and four carbons, with pauses to pass around the copies and let everyone catch up. The group then began to use a TRS-80 computer operated by sign language interpreters, who typed as best they could, which allowed all the participants to read the discussion on the computer display.

British MP JackAshley began experimenting with Palantype (British court reporting) in the 1970s.[25] In the 1983–4 academic year, court reporting was used in the United States for a seminar at Gallaudet University.[26] In 1989, ALDA began a partnership with the National Court Reporters Association (NCRA). NCRA now offers certification in real-time reporting. Many court reporters offer services to self-help meetings on a pro bono basis. Real-time reporting is now considered an access service under the Americans with Disabilities Act.

> I used real-time transcription to survive my PhD, both the research and the oral examination. For the research, I needed to interview a sample of people who could not sign. Using an interpreter would have interfered with taking accurate notes. I was able to set up Remote Real-time Reporting (I call it RRR) using two telephone lines, a computer at each end, and a reporter listening to my interviews through a microphone set up in my lab. Not only did I get accurate real-time transcription, but my interviews were already transcribed on disk for immediate analysis – a big advantage over audiotape. The remote technique is used regularly for television captioning and for transcribing speeches to large audiences. I'm the only person I know who has used RRR on a 'solitary' basis, yet obviously it has a great deal of potential, especially for clients without access to skilled local reporters.
>
> K.W.

It hasn't yet been standardized just who can provide these transcription services – indeed, it hasn't even been standardized what to call them. Sophisticated Americans call them 'CART' reporters (communication access real-time translation, formerly computer assisted real-time translation). The NCRA calls them certified real-time reporters (CRRs). We've seen a plethora of other terms, including 'notetaker,' 'typist,' 'captionist,' and 'real-time writer,' and we've toyed with the term 'print interpreter' to recognize their functional role as interpreters in communication settings.

4.5.1 *Primer on Real-Time Transcription*

There are three main forms that transcription can take: computer-assisted stenography (the good), computerized notetaking (the bad), and handwritten notetaking (the ugly).

Let's waste no time discussing handwritten notes. Pencil and paper function quite well between two people, but do nothing useful for the one deafened person in a group. With handwritten notes, the deafened person knows the general topics the others are talking about – approximately two topics after they have moved on. Access is not provided by making sure the deafened person knows 'they are talking about the budget now.' Rather, access is knowing exactly what is being said about the budget. Access is being able to join in the conversation and contribute. It is far more cost-effective to read the minutes of meetings than to waste time sitting through them while somebody else writes headlines on a notepad.

4.5.1.1 Computerized Notetaking

Computerized notetaking (also called computer-assisted notetaking, or CAN, or various proprietary names) uses standard word processing software to which various abbreviation-expanding macros have been added. The theory is that using standardized software will maximize the pool of operators (ideally volunteers) and minimize the specialized training required. (What training these 'notetakers' do receive is mostly just in the operation of their rig.)

> Pardon me for being unexcited by the prospect of having what I 'hear' and don't 'hear' determined by a person whose chief merit is her (or his) minimal but universal and thus cheaply available skills.
>
> K.W.

Computerized notetaking can be very useful for those hard-of-hearing and oral-deaf consumers who can participate in events through lipreading or oral interpreters. In these situations, the notetaker is not acting as an interpreter. These consumers merely want notes taken, because they can't take notes and lipread simultaneously. However, many deafened adults depend on transcriptions to comprehend and participate in events as they take place.

People can't type as fast as other people can speak, so a typist always ends up falling behind, abbreviating shamelessly, or getting utterly lost. The quandary is worst when a deafened adult requires transcription in the Real World. Bring a laptop and word processing software into a business meeting and everyone thinks you're all fixed up and ready to go. Unfortunately, depending on the skill and judgment of the operator, you either get just the bits they think were important (euphemistically called 'operator summarization'), or lag way behind, or continually interrupt the meeting to 'slow down please,' or all of the above. You spend much of your time mentally unjumbling the typos the typist has no time to backspace and correct, and while you're distracted from the content by that, the notetaker is committing further censorship. Operator summarization is the greatest assault that computerized notetaking commits on true access.

To the notetaker, who has no expertise in the specific domain of the meeting or event, and who is trying desperately to keep up, some words may seem superfluous though actually they are critical. Adjectives and other words of modification and emphasis often convey more than the subject-verb-object, yet these are the first words to go in notetaking. Print already lacks the vocal inflections and intonations that often convey important content. Without the adjectives, intonations, and digressions, the deafened adult reading print may quite easily form an inaccurate impression of what people are really saying. If these nuances are not essential in the business and higher education settings in which computerized notetaking is presently being touted, we can't imagine where they would be!

A few business users of computerized notetaking defend it. These people seem to share one common trait: they all have a regular operator, usually their secretary, who does have domain knowledge in addition to high-speed typing skills. It isn't fair for agencies to cite these unrepresentative cases in support of this approach, and it is unhelpful for these consumers to contradict the consumer majority. Most consumers will call an agency and will get someone they have never seen before, who may or may not have a professional demeanour appropriate to the situation, and who may or may not remember where all the function keys are.

In an all-deafened group, everyone is a user of the product, so there is no disadvantage to being dependent on this limited form of transcription. However, computerized notetaking even for self-help support groups has become much less desirable since the explosion in good-quality pro bono real-time reporting.

Even at its best, computerized notetaking never gives the nuances of language; when you see your own utterances on the screen, it makes you want to give up English and just grunt Neanderthalese. In English, we couch our words with adjectives and modifying phrases to soften or emphasize points we want to make. Someone says, 'Whaddya think about ordering some dinner now? Maybe there won't be a hearing person around to hear the doorbell when the delivery man arrives.' For this, the notetaker may transcribe, 'Haven't eaten, order dinner now.' A reasoned argument and quest for consensus becomes a dictate, and interpersonal misunderstandings ensue.

With all due respect to those of us we are describing, deafened people who rely on computerized notetaking can appear slow-witted, inattentive, rude, or simply passive, and this can be entirely a result of the notes they were reading. Usually these users are unaware of the poor impression they are making because they have no idea how badly censored the notes actually are.

> I find it degrading to misunderstand due to summarized, inadequate, or slow notes. If I am going to humiliate myself asking a stupid question, I want it to be my own stupid fault – and I want to be aware that I have humiliated myself.
>
> K.W.

4.5.1.2 Real-Time Court Reporting

The superior option is a real-time reporter, that is, a qualified court reporter (stenographer) with advanced qualifications in real-time reporting (CRR). Real-time court reporting is most commonly used for captioning live television news and sports programs; occasionally it is used in meetings of deaf/deafened people. With real-time reporting, the key is to prepare the vocabulary carefully in advance. This is because the reporter, instead of typing letter by letter, types the speech one syllable at a time using steno language key combinations on a special keyboard. The computer then recognizes the words from the syllable sequences. If a particular sequence of syllables, with the corresponding word, is not in the computer's dictionary, the word will not be decoded correctly and another word or combination of words with the same syllables will appear instead. For instance, after his seventh no-hitter Nolan Ryan was captioned a 'pitch whore' (/pitch/-/er/ in syllables). Admittedly, this may have been a keying error. Poor preparation of the translation dictionary likely accounts for those times when the names of both teams and their cities are displayed in various incorrect ways for the full duration of a ball game, or 'cochlear implant' – a popular topic among deafened people – being captioned 'cock leer implant' at a forum on the subject. If the wrong word comes up, the results can be mirth, or distraction, or anything in between: only a clairvoyant could have understood what was transpiring during the Gulf War on the basis of the Big Three U.S. networks' captions. In the 1990s, through a concerted effort, many real-time reporters worked hard to improve their skills, and nowadays they can produce excellent real-time transcriptions. Only computer-assisted, real-time court stenography technology can keep up with the pace of human speech and even approach giving deafened adults access to the Real World. It must be the standard for real-time transcription.

A shortage of providers of the service is a significant barrier. In its consumer information brochure, a major deaf services agency – one that arranges bookings for both computerized notetaking and real-time services – acknowledged the high quality of computer-assisted real-time stenography, but added that 'the costs are prohibitive.' Unfortunately, both the government and the business community perceive these agencies as advocates for consumers, and this gives others carte blanche to opt out of the appropriate standard of service. No one would dare to suggest the equivalent – that a few volunteers be trained in fingerspelling and sent out instead of sign language interpreters, because 'certified interpreters are expensive'; yet the agency has expended considerable effort advocating laptop word processing to the many institutions serving consumers who need real-time transcription. By providing mostly notetaking services, the agency also prevents consumers from becoming aware of real-time reporting. Consumers who have never seen real-time reporting may well be pleased to see computerized notetaking, because they have no idea what they are missing.

Our own behaviour as deafened people contributes to our ignorance of the possibilities. Because we can speak, we manage to be outwardly 'normal.' Because we accept the Hearing culture's stigma of deafness, we often withdraw from communication problems, instead of drawing attention to our needs and demanding solutions.

As long as the demand for real-time reporting is suppressed, few court reporters will acquire the advanced qualifications required for interpreting. Where are the jobs that make it worthwhile to leave the courtrooms?

Before one can evaluate these alternatives for transcription, one must have a mental image of the concept of 'access.' The common presumption is that 'anything is better than nothing' – that any form of transcription is access enough. We argue that the 'bad' and 'ugly' forms are harmful because they satisfy the *desire* to provide the service without actually providing it. The provider thinks the problem has gone away. ('Look! There's the notetaker sitting there!') Although a laptop and a temporary agency typist may be cheaper than a court reporter with real-time skills, the investment in the service is wasted unless the deafened consumer can participate as fully as if he or she were hearing the proceedings. Transcription should not intrude and stifle the consumer's full expression; it should convey spoken utterances with as many nuances as can be conveyed by printed language; and it should keep the deafened person up to the current topic of discussion.

4.6 Self-Help

Increasingly, medical experts are recognizing the significance of emotions and mental health to physical health. Self-help is valuable because it enhances emotional health by rebuilding positive support systems, not just because it offers instrumental benefits (e.g., learning about assistive devices and techniques).

We acknowledge that the term 'self-help' has different usages. In this book, we subscribe to the philosophy that self-help is a process *within the individual* that occurs in a supportive environment. We exclude the definition of self-help as a grassroots program of fundraising or boosterism in support of professional services or research. We also do not consider it self-help merely to remove professionals from providing advice about disease or disability management.

In self-help, there is no prescribed norm and no therapy agenda; nor are there any externally imposed expectations of any particular form of progress. In the self-help process, the individual, in a supportive environment, learns and grows and makes his own choices at his own pace. This philosophy seems permissive at first glance; yet following it can be even more complicated than applying an advanced professional knowledge base and expert techniques. Professional services are based on problem solving for individual clients. The professional has the responsibility to diagnose illness, relieve the condition, and refer the client as necessary to remedial assistance. The expertise resides in the professional, and the client – to a greater or lesser degree – is expected to defer to this expertise. For example, an otologist will expect the client's complete trust in his techniques of ear surgery. A social worker's client may have more self-determination, but the social worker still expects at least a commitment from the client as part of the therapy contract. Having elected to seek help from a professional, and having determined that the professional possesses the appropriate qualifications, the client does not expect the professional to earn trust by sharing her experiences and feelings. This clarity in the helping relationship simplifies the helping process, although of course it also requires the professional to acquire extensive education and training. Self-help requires no special knowledge base, but the self-help group must earn the members' trust before it can provide the supportive environment that is so essential to growth.

The self-help group's expertise resides not in one individual but rather in the collective knowledge and experience of the group. Among others who share their condition, people who struggle with feelings that they are defective can gain a sense of being normal. In the 'quid pro quo' environment, people who have difficulty confronting their emotions can admit those emotions.

In this chapter on professional help, we discuss self-help because the professional has a role to play in making referrals and possibly facilitating self-help support groups. People with more social support, of the sort they find in self-help groups, are more likely to seek information and follow recommendations. In that way, self-help often can compliment professional help.[27] Because there is no professional 'healer figure' in the group environment, participating in a group can sometimes nudge an overly dependent client into taking some responsibility for her own growth and healing.

People seek out experts for information about what happened biologically; they seek peer and self-help for the broader, persistent issues of what to do and how to cope.[28] 'One component of the effective interventions is dealing directly with emotional distress associated with fears regarding disease progression.'[29] 'One of the most important needs women have 9 months after [breast cancer] surgery is to understand what happened to them during surgery and why.'[30] For a time, as with hearing loss, biology is the source of the betrayal, and consequently the locus of the explanation. Elderly women accessing an Internet-based support for breast cancer could access professional help and peer/self-help. Discussion groups (peer) received twice as many uses (page views lasting longer than 1 minute) as 'Ask an expert' (33.9 per cent versus 17.1 per cent). Of the 20.4 per cent of uses involving question-and-answer and fact sheet material, most were related to cause and treatment.[31] Those answers are finite and often unsatisfactory for answering the underlying need: 'What happened to me? *Why* did it happen to me?' Although they cannot answer than question, peers reporting their own experiences are the most sought-after sources of insight.

Referrals to self-help should *not* be made for clients who lack an adequate sense of personal boundaries or who need professional help to deal with mental illness or other serious problems. Self-help is for clients whose difficulties are in the 'normal' range of responses to their condition, and who are ready to grow.

Provided that the person is mentally healthy and wants to grow, participation in self-help should begin as early as possible.[32] Exposure to peers can help relieve the initial 'peak devastation' of the diagnosis, and help the person process medical information and advice in making judgments about treatments. However, support groups are still valuable for ongoing coping, no matter how delayed the introduction. Studies have shown high levels of perceived value and satisfaction even when the first access was later – too late, say, for support in choosing treatments.[33] Even today, well into identity synthesis (we think), we still encounter situations that propel us into apoplexy, and feelings of utter frustration over the circumstance of deafness. For us as for others, support groups and self-help are never too late to be useful.

There is no role for a professional in the group; even so, for practical reasons it needs a leader-facilitator. A self-help group leader should be a member of the group. It doesn't hurt for that person to have training in a human services field, but it is better for the leader to be a deafened nonprofessional than a hearing social worker or counsellor. Especially in the early stages of coping, deafened people need every possible symbol of optimism and empowerment. Having a hearing professional leading the group symbolizes that 'we can't even discuss our own feelings without a hearing person to help us.' Don't dismiss the importance of symbols – if people are fragile enough to need self-help and support, little things like this can be profound.

The problem is, it may be the counsellor who first sees the need, not a deafened person. Only a tiny fraction of deafened people will even be aware that there can be groups for deafened people, and in many areas that tiny fraction may be made up of ... no one else.

Not wanting to start up with a professional-led group, but wanting to facilitate the mutual aid process, the professional may take a graduated approach. The professional begins by identifying the potential participants; she then plans an alternative function – perhaps a party or a seminar – to bring them together. These individuals can then be offered training in self-help, delivered by available trainers or suitable outside consultants. Bringing the group together, offering training, and providing an infrastructure (meeting place, communication access) is about all the professional can do until a group of deafened adults decide that they are ready and interested in growing and learning. Once the people have had a few chances to meet one another, they may request or at least be responsive to some help in starting a self-help program.

The following chapters provide information on peer help (educational and social programming) and self-help support groups for deafened people. These chapters are written for the deafened reader. We hope that professionals will find them useful for their content as well as for helping deafened clients understand the techniques.

PART TWO

Support

Chapter 5

Peer Help

Peer help is the territory between professional help and self-help, where organized group activities other than self-help enable deafened people to meet and learn from one another. In the peer help environment, deafened people themselves – not professionals – take charge. Because peers have the same experience, being deafened, they can provide insights that a hearing person with extensive professional training may not have. But it is a little like comparing the bird's-eye view with the bug's-eye view: the birds don't really know what it is like down there on the ground, for the bugs who are unable to fly. If you want to know about the immediate living conditions of bugs, you ask a bug. However, a bug isn't versed in the survival needs of all the different kinds of bugs, nor can it see what lies in the next furrow. One kind of bug might be better off staying in the present furrow in a rainwater puddle; another might be better off moving on, because the next furrow has a clump of buttercups in it. Removing professionals from the process of giving advice doesn't automatically make the advice wiser or more accurate. Peers should not start prescribing 'right' and 'wrong' things to do.

This chapter explains peer help activities such as educational sessions, socials, and mini-conferences. It also discusses the value of special interest groups and outlines the unique ALDA-con phenomenon. Finally, it covers leadership and administrative issues that often arise when peer help and self-help push or pull deafened people toward forming an organized association.

5.1 Educational Sessions

Educational sessions serve a useful double-function. Some deaf-ened people, especially newcomers, may be skittish about just point-blank signing up for a self-help support group series. They may be afraid that everyone else knows each other, and wonder what they themselves could possibly have to say, and just generally be afraid of the unknown. Some deafened people are struggling with a world in which much of everything is hard to understand. Educational sessions are good 'excuses' for those who are trying to convince themselves to face the unfamiliar. They can sneak into the room, sit at the back, invisibly absorb some expert's information, and leave quietly – but elevated. They can persuade significant others to accompany them to jointly learn a little about this condition that is affecting them both, in different ways.

The disadvantage is that educational sessions very often set up a professional as the 'expert' on the condition that we are liv-ing with and that she is not. This undermines our confidence that we know our own experience; it also primes us to simply accept what we are told to do. Peer-help program planners should plan their educational sessions with care to make them the marketing tools and empowering experiences they should be.

An 'expert' should be framed on your program within a value structure that has been chosen by the peer-led organizing group, not defined and imparted by the expert. 'Experts' should be invited to provide topic-specific information, not to be the font from which all wisdom flows. 'Expert' opinion should be coun-terbalanced by deafened people's experiences, both good and bad, with the topic. Ample discussion and question-and-answer should enable the audience to go home with information they desired; in the same vein, the 'experts' should leave having learned something too. Table 5.1 provides some example topics and program outlines that illustrate these principles.

Establishing the expressed and implied value structure is a delicate matter that goes beyond mere politics and public rela-

TABLE 5.1
Complementing 'experts' on example educational session programs

Cochlear implant

Doctor: how it works, how surgery is done	Audiologist: how candidates are evaluated, how rehabilitation is done	Panel of users to describe briefly good and bad experiences (when inviting, make sure panel is balanced)	Ample discussion, question/answer

Television captioning or telephone relay service

Manager or engineer: how the system works, who provides the service, how they are trained	Demonstration, live or on video	Knowledgeable deafened people: areas of strengths and weaknesses in the current service, where it should go	Ample discussion, question/answer

New disability rights regulations

Lawyer, regulator: what the proposed (or new) laws are, where they apply and who will benefit, when they will come into force	Disability rights activist/advocate: how the larger disabled community feels about the laws, and how individual consumers can make the best of it	Deafened leaders: specific provisions and omissions that pertain to the special case of deafened people	Ample discussion, question/answer

tions and touches the very heart of the adjustment process. People who find a particular value structure offensive will be deterred from further involvement. One value that arises in many educational programs is the Holy Grail of *curing* deafness. Although many people desire it, to promote 'the cure' as the Holy Grail leaves most people empty-handed and perpetually disappointed. The idea of a cure has a strong appeal for some people in the very early stages of adjustment, but it equally strongly offends people who have satisfied themselves that there is no viable cure and who want to move on. The resulting polarization can work against attempts to find common ground within the group to support a self-help process.

The 'cure' theme offers a few temptations. Call to mind for a moment the controversial celebrity telethons and direct mail fundraising campaigns that play on pathetic children in need of help. Educational programs that portray deafened people in this light tend to attract more attention and support (especially money) from external sources. People who are in the *identity comparison* stage of adjustment have a high outward energy level that they are ready to mobilize in the search for a 'cure' (see the Model of Deafened Adjustment in Section 2.4); people in the later *identity concession* and *identity recognition* stages of adjustment are directing relatively more of their energy at introspection. Unfortunately, the implication that the deafened person is defective until cured is fundamentally intolerable to those who have progressed from *identity recognition* to *activism* and beyond. What is happening here is that the very key to stimulating enthusiasm for the program is turning off the people who have reached the more advanced stages of adjustment and who have so much to offer in terms of peer support.

Equally risky is the pro–Deaf Culture theme, which some people find utterly terrifying. We have read letters from deafened people who find any suggestion that we are in any way 'like them' to be absolutely odious, but there may be a majority who would enjoy such programs as long as the comparisons were gently drawn. For instance, a program that focused on how a 'non-native' deaf person could enjoy Deaf poetry and theatre might be easier to swallow.

Other educational sessions do not require 'experts.' Panels of deafened people can discuss particular topics of wide interest: marriage and relationships, parenting, job changing. Once again, ample provision for audience participation helps make these sessions dynamic. Avoid setting up some of the deafened group members as experts or role models. This can hinder their own adjustment and create dysfunctional dependencies. Peers help best by being peers, not by being 'big brothers' or guides.

Marketing sessions and demonstrations of technical devices are dubious 'educational programs' and are probably best presented in an 'information fair' context, for instance, at an exhibit table during an educational forum on another topic. The audience will be at many different levels of familiarity with assistive devices, and the people who already have a bunch of devices are not going to be that interested in a demonstration of, say, how a vibrating alarm clock works. It jeopardizes the group's objectivity to be treated as a marketing target for purveyors of new gadgets. But it can be useful to offer these items as exhibits during a session with another theme. Other similar retail/display materials that make a nice complement to educational sessions are books on all topics related to deafness, and sign language trinkets (jewellery, clothing, ornaments, and knick-knacks). These are difficult to find in mainstream book and gift stores, and inviting vendors to exhibit them is a convenience for deafened people who do not know where else to find them.[1] Despite varying familiarity with sign language, deafened people often collect this paraphernalia and reading material the way tourists collect mementos.

5.2 Socials

Socials are a real challenge. You send out survey after survey and people check off that they want bowling and board games, and month after month no one shows up. Yet the people who go to self-help seem to love chatting at coffee break time so much so that it's hard to get them back into the group for the second half. Our guess is that the sharing in self-help is the prerequisite that makes the social affinity happen: by the time people have an hour of honesty behind them, they feel like real friends. Receiving an invitation to a bowling party of deafened strangers and acquaintances just doesn't feel the same. Many people just dread socials. More introverted people may simply skip them, even though they wish for some kind of a social life – that they could shake the fear and go. An entirely social group is therefore a 'hit or miss' proposition. Everything depends on the people involved.

Some groups, like the famous Chicago chapter of ALDA, thrive in their socials. A great deal depends on the similarity of people and their tastes, so it's likely that if everyone really likes raucous BYOB/pot luck parties in a basically WASP ambience, and that is what you are offering, you'll get good attendance.

Having a core self-help group helps create strong friendships that will help fuel a party, and a good party may relax people enough to sign up for a future self-help series.

A difficulty with a cohesive social group is that eventually the starvation for social affiliation is satisfied. The group members have become genuine friends beyond the group and its official events. They have resolved the profound loneliness they brought with them on first arrival in the group. They now attend social events not out of a need to fill the emptiness, but rather from a desire to see existing friends.The group that becomes old friends must guard against shutting out newcomers (see Section 6.5, 'Recruitment and Outreach').

5.3 The Mini-Conference

When you don't have much of a track record with the people you want to involve, you may have a hard time determining what will appeal to people. One approach is to try to be all things to everyone and combine both educational and social activities in a mini-conference. A mini-conference is a good use of time when you're attempting to involve people over a large geographic area. Infrequent travel makes longer distances less burdensome, and a longer program makes the trip more worthwhile.

To put together a mini-conference, you could schedule a late afternoon educational session with a suitable topic and presenters, invite interesting exhibitors (potentially to sponsor the event), set up self-help program registration at the exhibit desk (with take-home flyers available for people who can't commit on the spot), and plan a social event over dinner. Table 5.2 provides a model organization that can be divided up among a group of interested volunteer organizers, or handled by a professional with clerical help. There are infinite possible modifications to the timing and topics; this starting point is provided to help those who don't know where else to begin.

Invite professionals, and encourage them to publicize the event to deafened people you don't know yet. Hint about – or

TABLE 5.2
Sample organization for a mini-conference

Model half-day program		Co-ordinators (some tasks could be combined)
1:00	Registration and exhibits	• Educational program:
2:00–3:15	Educational session	– invite presenters, greet and guide them on-site, introduce them, moderate sessions
3:15–3:45	Break, exhibits, beverages	– determine the amount and type of audiovisual equipment required by
3:45–5:00	Educational session continues	presenters and communication access, and order it
5:00	Dinner buffet, pizza, etc.	• Communication access (arrange real-time transcription and interpreting and
evening	Party activity (if attendance seems likely to support it) such as karaoke, trip to captioned film, etc.	microphone)
		• Exhibitor recruitment and liaison
		• Sponsors (may combine with exhibit co-ordinator) (raise enough money to pay for costs not covered by registration fees)
		• Refreshments and buffet
		• Publicity
Refer to Table 5.1 for some program details.		• Advance registration (if any), nametags, discreetly assist those who cannot afford to pay the announced registration fee
		• Treasurer (keep clear, open accounts)
		• Registration/information for next self-help series (self-help leader if possible)
		Liaison with the facility could be taken on by the program co-ordinator or the exhibit co-ordinator. Most facilities prefer a sole liaison person (reserving rooms, requesting furniture set-ups, ordering audiovisual equipment, and deciding catering if any)

ask outright for – financial sponsorships to cover food and beverages. You can collect a small fee for food and beverages at the door, but try to be prepared to subsidize those in real financial hardship. Don't forget nametags: nobody can lipread names.

When a group is secure and an open event doesn't need to be all things to all people, single-purpose events can succeed: the summer picnic, the Hallowe'en party, the theatre trip, the guest lecture. Even for these groups, a 'mini-conference' has its uses as a forum for reaching out to new people, and as an annual celebration of the value of the group.

5.4 Special Interest Groups

Becoming deaf is not a free pass to escape the other problems and issues of life. It seems that many people have a mental image that every person has only one problem; partly for this reason, programs and groups often fail to deal with multiple challenges. Sometimes the problem results from deafness: as a result of the social isolation that many deafened people experience, dysfunctional responses such as chemical dependency are common. In other cases, deafness interferes with getting effective treatment because existing services and facilities are not accessible, or are only accessible to deaf people who are fluent sign language users, so people who already had a substance abuse problem have nowhere to turn. We have had a huge response at deafened gatherings to organized 'recovery' theme self-help sessions. We believe there are many other special interests.

Some deafened people feel doubly marginalized due to their sexual identity; others struggle with single parenting on top of deafness; still others have additional disabilities. As well, some have a certain type of career and will not be able to visualize adjusting within their professional lives without the example and support of deafened people in the same field. Often, the only person who can really give the needed support is someone who shares *all* of the significant characteristics, not just the deafness characteristic. We strongly advocate special interest groups within deafened groups. Some sorts of special interests will be fairly thinly dispersed, so that sharing among those with that special interest is likely to take place on the Internet, through newsletters, or at infrequent gatherings. Members who have particular needs on top of late deafness should be encouraged to find or start a special interest group, rather than dissuaded from doing so. We see no 'threat' to the main group – if anything, we predict it will *increase* the sense of affiliation, because accommodating the special interest is symbolic of accepting the whole person. The special interest group itself can determine whether its activities will consist of socials, self-help, or other options.

5.5 ALDAcon

ALDA held a free leadership workshop in October 1989. This was the event that later became known as ALDAcon. It was attended by forty-one Americans and one Canadian. ALDAcon has been held annually ever since (though no longer free).

ALDAcon workshops run the gamut, and typically include the following:

- Self-help sessions (which run throughout the convention)
- Sessions on using telephone relay services, cochlear implants, and other deafness-related topics
- Sign language basic training
- Lifestyle sessions about activities that are generally inaccessible to deaf people in the typical hometown (e.g., ballroom dancing, Tai Chi)

Sessions on relationships are always popular, as many deafened people struggle to redefine relationships with hearing partners, work colleagues, and their family of origin. Families are encouraged to attend the conferences. In recent years, many workshops have featured panels on which deafened people discuss how they have dealt with a particular challenge, whether it is addiction or parenthood. Self-help leadership training and support group sessions have been offered at almost every convention. (The self-help principles promoted by ALDA are closely compatible with the methods described in Chapter 6.)

In addition to self-help training, several ALDAcon traditions have taken root. The buddy program ensures that newcomers can always count on someone to help them break the ice and feel at home. A karaoke soirée provides an opportunity to screech off-key some fondly remembered tunes, some of which have become ALDA anthems ('Jeremiah was a bullfrog / He was a good friend of mine / I never understood a single word he said ...') Meals are an important part of the ALDAcon program because so much of the candid sharing, bonding, and learning takes place while trying to figure out whether the waiter is offering coffee or tea ('and

by the way, how do you communicate when people have a foreign accent?'). Many participants report that their first ALDAcon
exposure was a life-altering experience.

5.6 Formal Leadership and Governance

A formal organization is entirely different from a self-help group
or a committee planning an educational program. There is a benefit to having an organization, in that it offers more self-determination than deferring to a professional or agency to brings
events together. For deafened people, successfully organizing a
group or event is a source of pride and esteem: it can reassure
them that they have abilities even if they can't hear. There are
many reference books available for starting and running non-
profit organizations, and we do not intend to repeat the general
guidelines for organizational leadership. After comparing those
general principles with our own experiences in deafened groups
and other management/committee roles, we have made a few
observations, which are outlined below.

Organize to suit your particular motley crew. There is no reason why the steering committee, board, council, executive, or
whatever it calls itself has to have any particular set of position
titles with one person per spot. As long as any money the group
acquires is handled appropriately and openly, and is properly
documented, we advocate letting the leadership structure arise
from available talents until the size of the group provides
enough options for elections to a more conventional roster of
positions. The group absolutely must conduct regular (i.e.,
annual) elections to determine who should be the nominal
leader, chairperson, president, emperor, or whatever title you
choose. No group should have to remain under the thumb of the
person who had the idea first. When people resign their positions – and invariably, some eventually will, because the people
involved are inherently in a volatile stage of their lives – the
group needs to accept those resignations graciously and without
prejudice. That way, those people may be open to returning
when the troubles pass. Wheedling and concerted flattery may

entice a person back into his role out of sheer guilt, but it may not be the best thing for him from a self-help perspective, and it may adversely affect him and possibly the group. The administrative contact person doesn't have to be the person who leads the self-help sessions.

Pre-empt meddling and hurt feelings with mutual agreements. Nowhere is the alleged paranoia of deafness more evident than in the need for every member of the organizing group to discuss and have a say in every issue. We sometimes think that apparent paranoia is merely natural perceptiveness: people really *are* talking about you because you *are* peculiar by being deaf. However, the behaviour of nearly every deafened administrative group has made us suspect that there is more to it than that. Having been shut out intentionally or just for practical reasons from decisions in every other environment, deafened people seem starved for inclusion in decision making. To avoid conflicts down the road, a group needs to reach a consensus on what is 'due consultation' and 'checks and balances' and what is meddling. The group will be dependent on the good will of volunteers; even at the national and international levels, deafened groups have not been able to secure funding for paid staff. The only reward for volunteers is autonomy and the satisfaction of seeing the results of their work. Group leaders need to agree in advance to judge one another's contributions not by whether something could be *improved upon* but by whether that something *accomplishes the goal*. Stating goals clearly in advance is essential. The alternative is good-enough projects never implemented because someone thought they could be better, and attrition of volunteers. When enough time is spent on setting goals and a little willpower is applied, the good will and initiative of volunteers can be maintained, and accusations of micromanagement can be avoided.

Separate governance from self-help. People often hide behind administrative issues. Groups can fritter away meeting after meeting discussing what it should call itself, how it should decide when meetings or events will be held, how various reporting channels will work, and whether it should co-operate with some other group or agency on a proposed project or joint

activity. These petty deliberations are not entirely due to paranoia: tying up the agenda with administrative issues is a way to
avoid self-help discussions that some people find uncomfortable
(or in their expressed opinion, unnecessary). If what you really
want is self-help, consider whether you really *need* to form a
club, association, chapter, or other organized activity.

Let people determine their own ambitions. We can't criticize
the pursuit and exercise of organizational power, because it is
natural and at least it is the choice of the person involved. Unfortunately, we may be tempted to push someone *else* to take on a
particular office or task, for instance, because we think he needs
an opportunity to learn how strong he is. Self-help groups gain so
much insight into what motivates group members that it is possible to push the right buttons to get someone to do more than he
really feels comfortable doing. This is a misuse of the deep personal sharing of self-help. There could be good outcomes but
there are several bad outcomes. The group starts taking the person for granted, and dreading the constant pressure, the individual withdraws from all participation and cannot see the group as
a safe place to go for support. If and when he doesn't deliver, both
the organization and our relations with him suffer. (Bailing him
out and giving him credit can also backfire years later, when he
has gained in ambition but not necessarily in competence.)

Avoid becoming a personality cult. A charismatic leader can
help a fledgling group seem dynamic and attractive to newcomers. However, the whole group needs to understand the ideals
and remain true to them and not simply defer to the charismatic
leader's interpretation of the ideals. It is possible for organizational roles to spill out onto social relationships, and vice versa.
Leaders placed in the cult leader role may feel constrained from
showing weakness; conversely, they may feel obligated to continue demonstrating their struggle after they have actually fin-
ished working through it.

5.7 No Bad Members

A feeling that seems to simmer beneath the surface in some

groups is the idea that individual members or prospective members owe something to the group, such as attendance, participation, or organizational effort. Those who rarely attend or who do not contribute very much are sometimes considered bad members and referred to openly as 'phantoms' or freeloaders. From time to time, one of the more enthusiastic members will remark that most of the others reap the benefits while 'just a few of us seem to do all the work.' This particularly arises when the group undertakes additional activities and services such as a newsletter or social events.

5.7.1 Subscribers Are Not Members

This criticism of the 'phantom' names ignores the fact that many mailing list names were merely one-time contacts by people who never asked to be considered *members*. The mailing list person turned them into *subscribers* – perhaps against their will! Even willing subscribers are not members. *Membership* requires an active expression of intent to become a member: completing a membership application form and paying dues, or signing up for self-help.

Some people become subscribers after well-meaning neighbours or family members send in their names. Invariably, some unwitting subscribers are students who requested materials *once* for a school assignment and who never did have a long-term interest in the group. Also, names are sometimes added in an exchange of lists with another group. Finally, some names are of professionals, who are added by someone who thinks this may lead to referrals.

If there are no dues, the group has no mechanism for deleting a person who does not confirm his desire for membership with a payment. With all the other unwanted mail people receive, there is little chance that someone will bother to tell the group to stop sending an unwanted occasional newsletter. As long as printing and postage costs are not a concern (e.g., when these are subsidized by a sponsor or grant), this unbridled harvesting of names conveys a positive – albeit misleading – image of the group's growth to potential funding agencies who evaluate the importance of a program in terms of the volume of 'contacts' with consumers. The mailing list bloat may even have happened deliberately for this reason. When times are tight and no funding is forthcoming, the group would prefer to send newsletters only to those who want them. We speak from experience when we say it is far easier to differentiate from the outset than to sift through 2,500 names in search of some sign of each person's interest.

The group itself may confuse subscriptions with involvement in the decision-making process and feel obligated to send detailed rationales and ballots to all the people on the mailing list, allowing ample time for responses – perhaps even extending deadlines when the rate of return appears extremely low. Despite your regular mailing to 200 people, the ten who show up regularly may constitute the majority of those with any shred of ongoing interest.

5.7.2 Simple Mailing Records

These dilemmas reinforce our recommendation that the group set up its mailing list records carefully in the first place. Table 5.3 outlines a simple structure that can be set up on a computer.

Many groups initially decide not to make a distinction between deafened people and hearing supporters, in the belief that this is somehow discriminatory. However, making a distinction does not prevent the group from extending full privileges to members of every class. And unless a distinction is made, it is impossible for the group's organizers to keep a tally of the number of *deafened* people in its membership. Even if there are no major decisions that should be reserved for the deafened membership to make, it is helpful to have a register of the size of the deafened population, because it is informative when it comes time to make appeals for financial support and set targets for outreach.

It is better to avoid 'Mr and Mrs' member records; ultimately, the group wants to know the name of the *deafened* partner. If both members of a couple are deafened, both names could be

TABLE 5.3
Simple mailing list structure

Name and address	**Contact**
Information of one person	Date of the latest contact
(not couple)	(to flag likely obsoletes)
Classification	**Source**
Deafened, personal other,	You may want to record how
business other	member heard of the group
Mailing	**E-mail**
Yes if a subscriber; no if only	Record addresses in standard
a contact; no for deafened	Internet notation
spouse not wanting duplicate	
newsletter	
Expiration	**Phone**
Expiration of paid dues if dues	Record numbers in TTY, voice,
are charged; duration of 'trial	and fax categories for home
subscription' if these are given	and work (but only those
(after expiration, do not delete,	numbers that the member
just convert to 'non-mailing')	wishes listed)

registered separately, to tally the population, with one indicated as nonmailing, to avoid duplicate newsletters.

Among the non-deafened, those with business interests in deafness (professionals, agencies, vendors) might be distinguished from individuals with a merely personal interest (family members, friends, and so on). For one thing, it is easier to target businesses for scholarships or advertising sales if these are classified separately. You might wish to distinguish between vendors, professionals and agencies, and the media, or you might not, depending on the mailing subsets you want to create. You can always add two separate groups into a subtotal, but if you don't capture the differences in the first place, you can never tally them separately. You can still treat them to the identical membership privileges as long as you want to.

If avoiding wasted postage and nuisance mail is a goal, people who request information or sample newsletters should be sent what they have requested but should not be added in perpetuity. These people are 'contacts,' and it is legitimate for the group to note having made contact with them when it comes time to assess impact on the community. However, it is inefficient to convert those contacts into subscribers or to consider them members. The contact name should be entered and coded as 'non-mailing,' and no further newsletters should be sent. Once in a while it may be useful to have the names and addresses of formerly interested people – for example, when soliciting funds or announcing conferences.

Occasionally, the group will receive the name of a deafened person who is not ready to sign up and become a member, especially if that entails filling in a membership form that says in black and white, 'I am deaf from now on.' Our philosophy is to send mailings to these people as long as it is financially sustainable. They may need to feel support before they are ready to request it. If it is not sustainable to send them mailings, a 'trial subscription' can be given to them, for perhaps two or three newsletters, to let them know that the group is there if they need it. Also, they can be sent a notice if the group changes its mailing address, so they always know where to find the group at such time as they become ready.

Obviously, increased sophistication – and complexity – can be added. For instance, flags can be added to indicate those who do not wish to be listed in a directory or included on a list sold or exchanged with another group, or those who would rather not have their name given to new members. Fields could be added to record virtually unlimited sorts of voluntary information: type of deafness, career and family information, interest in working on committees, special interest group membership, past and current registration in self-help series, and so on.

This simple structure can meet the most basic needs by having the computer produce subsets of the entire list for different purposes:

- A tally of deafened people can be made by requesting a list of all the names (contacts, subscribers, and members) with the 'deafened' classification.

- Potential self-help meeting locations can be eliminated if they are obviously a long way from most of the deafened people's postal codes.
- Mailing labels for newsletters can be produced for those with 'yes' in the mailing field and a future expiration date.
- Reminders for dues can be sent to those whose expiration dates are past or imminent.
- Appeals for financial sponsorship can be sent to all the names on the list, or perhaps just to the business agencies and to professionals.
- Businesses and agencies can be invited to purchase advertising.
- Notices of upcoming self-help sessions can be sent to all deafened people.
- Ballots for voting can be sent to deafened people and anyone whose dues (if applicable) are paid up.

Last-contact dates suggest whether the addresses are still current; they are also searchable for producing a record of how many contacts the group received within the past year, which comes in handy at grant-seeking time. Organizers can consider removing names if the person is not deafened, has not paid current dues, and has not had a recent contact.

5.7.3 No Strings Attached to Self-Help Membership

There is a fine line between a self-help group and a club, association, or chapter. In a self-help setting, there is no obligation whatsoever other than what is covered in the group's ground rules. It is completely fair for any member to sign up for the occasional series, and even to participate minimally. As long as he or she is honest and fulfils the commitment to attending the sessions in the series, and does not violate other rules, the members who take all the chores of group leading and newsletter editing have no grounds for complaint.

Not signing up for self-help sessions, and not volunteering to organize socials or contribute to the newsletter, and rarely attending functions, does not make a person a 'bad member.' Under the self-help philosophy, *people help themselves as and when they are ready*. Someone who receives the newsletter and otherwise does nothing else is either not yet ready to do more, or adequately helped by just doing that.

Those who undertake additional roles must do so out of a desire to help *themselves*. Anyone who joins a self-help group to help *others* is off to an inauspicious start and must make a serious appraisal of his own needs and values. It is inappropriate to expect to be able to set a standard of service and have others accept and meet it: this only leads to disappointment and disagreement. The problem is not in the activity that the 'eager beaver' takes on, but in the expectations for how others will respond. If the activity itself is something the person wants to do, and if there is no expectation that other members of the group will reciprocate in a particular way, then the activity is valid and worthwhile. It must be genuinely performed for its own intrinsic enjoyment. We strongly discourage any expectations of return on this effort, and that includes expectations of receiving recognition, inspiring others to perform commensurate activity, and so on. From personal experience, we have found that we truly feel helped by writing for fellow members (newsletters, website). And because we have been willing to continue doing so with no strings attached, it has been enormously rewarding.

Chapter 6

Self-Help

There are a variety of ways to define 'self-help.' In our definition, self-help means *we each help ourselves, as and when we are ready.* Other people may use the term to describe a grassroots program of fundraising,[1] or boosterism in support of professional services or research, or having other deaf people instead of professionals providing advice about coping and management of deafness. In our experience, the self-help work that deafened people most need is within themselves.

If we are each helping ourselves, why do we even need a group? Groups offer many benefits for people working through challenges like becoming deaf. Foremost among these is the sense of support encountered in an environment in which the members trust and care about one another. You are the only person who can know what is best for you, but this doesn't mean you're alone. The second benefit is that all of the other group members are deafened. Members can feel 'normal' for that characteristic, and not different, as they may feel in their everyday environment surrounded by people who can hear. Groups provide a mosaic of personal backgrounds and experiences, and the members can compare those experiences in the context of other similarities and differences. This can lead to new things to try and new ways to think about feelings. In the honesty and sharing of the self-help group, members model for one another the emotional coping skills they use, and succeed – and fail – with, and each member can learn from the experiences of the others.

Positive Aspects of Self-Help Groups
- Members gain facts and knowledge about the experience.
- Members learn mechanisms of social coping from those who are successfully living with the condition.
- Members increase their motivation and receive support by communicating with others who are sharing a similar life experience.
- Members who model successful problem-solving behaviours provide reinforcement for both new and long-term members.
- Members are able to evaluate their own progress through feedback from other members, and through sharing their experiences with other members at various stages of the condition.
- Members are able to identify with the group, which provides a tangible sense of belonging, and which minimizes isolation and alienation.
- Members are able to help themselves by caring about others.

The emphasis is on emotional coping, although we also need to explain our practical coping so that people can put our emotional coping in perspective. There is little harm in someone who uses a TTY advising someone who would like to know how. There is also little growth if we remain at the level of device operation. To cope emotionally, we need to do our own work, not copy someone else's.

The fine line: We do help one another, but not by trying to give help. Others help us merely by sharing their honest descriptions of certain experiences and feelings, and we use this information to choose how we cope with similar experiences or handle our feelings about them.

In this chapter we discuss the following: open versus closed groups; group size; requirements for membership; recruitment and outreach; and the numerous details involved with the leader's preparation. Procedures for actually conducting group sessions, and the rules for the groups, are in the next chapter.

6.1 Group Format: Open or Closed

In the terminology of support groups, groups may be 'open' or closed.' Both open and closed groups have their merits. Our preferences are based on practical experience, and there is room for adapting to local conditions. Whether the group is open or closed affects some other aspects, such as recruitment, so we will discuss this first. (Whether the group is open or closed, it is only open to deafened people. See the rules and explanations about observers and visitors in Section 8.4.)

6.1.1 Open

An open group means that a newcomer – any deafened person – is welcome to attend any meeting. This means the group is 'there' for people who finally get over their resistance to seeking support. They may need to seize the moment lest they fall back between the cracks for a while. The problem is that with many groups, every time a new person comes the members go back to square one and give long introductions about themselves and the background of the group, and no actual progress is ever made. Because anyone can attend any time, for the first time or a long time since their last participation, the ground rules must be reviewed in detail at each session. Of course this eats into the group's time.

If the leader monitors the introduction business and if extra time is allowed so that the actual self-help time is adequate, an open group can work fine.

6.1.2 Closed

Closed groups aren't closed to everyone forever. They work like school courses, where you register and attend all the sessions for a term. Regular attendance is not such a burden when it is for a limited number of weeks. Members can expect a certain commitment of the fellow members to the group. Seeing the same people at each session leads to perceptions of 'safety' over the course of the series, which is valuable for self-help. When the set of sessions is over, the group takes a short break. Newcomers are welcome to sign up for the next set, and the old members can choose to sign up again. The first session covers the ground rules for the group, with just a short reminder at each meeting thereafter. The final session incorporates some 'saying goodbye,' to give some closure to the participants, as the group will probably change its composition for the next term.

6.1.3 What We Like

We think a good format is closed group, with sets of five or six sessions, one every two weeks for ten or twelve weeks, and with the members making a commitment to themselves and to one another to attend each session (see Figure 6.1). The group then takes a break for two to four weeks and starts a new set. This way there are four 'quarters' in a year. A social or deafness-related educational function open to interested people, past and potential members, and family and friends can be held during the break, where people can get information and sign up for the next series. We like weekly meetings, but it seems there are few places where the driving and parking time and expense aren't unreasonable. At present, there are few groups and they are scattered widely, so even a 'nearby' group may still be an hour from home. (A big city's population density isn't necessarily an advantage when commuting cross-town can take an hour.) If eight to ten people happen to live close together and prefer to meet weekly, we really encourage this. The terms can be shorter – say, weekly for six weeks, with four weeks off between terms. However, for most groups, getting the group size and serving the needs of those people in the outskirts means biweekly meetings.

We think monthly meetings are too infrequent to foster the bonding, trust, and commitment that a group needs. We have seen too many 'third Tuesday' efforts limp along, dying, or failing even while they still meet, because the group never

Figure 6.1: Quarterly closed support group calendar (example)

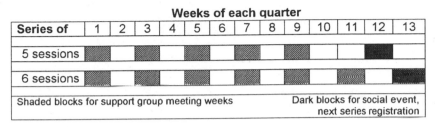

reached the level of familiarity and 'safety' that brings out sharing.

6.2 Group Size

Communication in groups of deafened people is slowed by the need for transcription. For the same amount of sharing as a similar group of hearing people, a group of deafened people either needs more time or fewer people. Since time is usually limited, the best group size will be smaller than suggested by generic self-help group guidelines.Whether the group is open or closed, eight to ten is a nice number. This allows the 'air time' for all to speak if they want, while including enough people to get a diverse sampling of how different people handle the same experiences. We encourage a group of even three people to go ahead and meet, but they should make a little effort to publicize the group so that other people will join in the future. If there are a dozen interested people, that size can work, especially if they are willing to spend a little longer at each meeting, but we encourage a group of, say, twenty to split into two groups for self-help purposes (and get both groups together for big socials!).

6.3 Membership

When you publicize the group among people who may refer participants, you should ensure that those professionals and agencies are aware of the group's nature – that is, what the group will and will not do for people, and what kind of people are appropriate to refer. Competent professionals and agencies will understand these principles, but you need to *tell them* what they are. You could organize a special presentation and meeting just to inform interested professionals about the group.

6.3.1 *Open to Healthy, Deafened Adults Who Want to Heal and Grow*

There is a big difference between professional counselling and self-help. A therapist is equipped to provide therapy to ill clients seeking to become well; self-help groups exist for normal people who feel pain and seek to heal and grow. Obviously, there is a fuzzy border between these. For example, depression can be considered a 'normal' response to becoming deaf; at the same time, deafened people can have some unrelated mental illness. The main thing to remember here is that the self-help group is not *expected* to provide therapy or solve individual problems.

For her own good and the good of the group, a person must have adequate boundaries to prevent sharing things she should keep private. People with weak boundaries may share information and later feel uncomfortable about it. An individual should be able to respect her own boundaries even with other people setting the example of sharing, or with someone asking for the information. Her boundaries must also limit her from sharing too much, and dumping too much information on the group beyond what is appropriate to the topic. The individual must respect the boundaries of others, not coercing individual sharing, and not advancing on another member during breaks or between sessions to offer advice, ask advice, commiserate, or seek details. Within the group procedure that we explain in the next chapter, a member may veto a topic if that topic would cause distress. People must have adequate boundaries to assert the veto privilege. People without adequate boundaries should not be referred or admitted to a self-help group until their boundaries are more secure.

Our boundaries tell us where we end and others begin. Healthy boundaries enable us to put others in perspective in our lives. When we join a group, we understand what it can do for us and what it cannot do for us – what we must do for ourselves. A person with healthy boundaries understands that he can expect others to adopt or respect certain behaviours (group rules, laws), but he cannot legislate, demand, or judge their attitudes.

With weak boundaries, we are threatened when others disagree with us and even when they choose paths that differ from our own. A person with weak boundaries expects that the group must eventually come around to his own views, because he cannot differentiate the group from himself. He will share everything with the group because he does not perceive any separation between his private knowledge and the group's knowledge. If the group disagrees with him, he may perpetuate the dispute, or suffer stress privately. Letting go of this distress requires him to develop generalized apathy.

With strong boundaries, we can maintain care and concern about ourselves while recognizing that others go their own way – even others in close groups to which we belong. We understand that our task is not to control the group but to put it in perspective.

Members must be prepared to respect and abide by the group's rules. Also, they must be in the group voluntarily with a desire to grow. They must be committed to the principles and beliefs of self-help and actively practise their new self-knowledge in their daily life. They must take responsibility for their own growth, and for making choices among alternatives.

6.3.2 Coerced and Involuntary Participants

It has happened that a counsellor from a rehabilitation or social assistance program requires a client to attend a self-help program as a condition of continuing services. Perhaps the thought is that the client is not taking enough personal interest in 'getting better,' whatever that means. The referral to the group may be parcelled with an outright threat of cutting services, or it may be a strong suggestion that a client who is fearful of authority follows unwillingly. Because the self-help group is not run by professionally trained counsellors or therapists, there is no safety valve for the more serious problems these people may bring. This person's participation has a different set of assumptions: people who voluntarily attend have made a choice to try to cope with deafness; people who have been coerced have not yet made that choice. A competent counsellor will not make this sort of referral other than through a misunderstanding. When such a person is sent to the group, the leader should contact the referring professional to review (or introduce) the group's principles and ground rules.

During registration for a closed group, newcomers should have been asked how they have come to be there. If they came through a referral, the name of the counsellor should be noted. Even if the person professes to be there voluntarily, problems may later arise that seem related to coercion. In that case, the group leader may wish to contact the counsellor to express her concerns. It may be necessary for the good of the group to withdraw the client from the group. The counsellor would then be responsible for any follow-up.

In an open group, you may not routinely know how a newcomer has been referred to the group. Possibly, the leader will have an opportunity to speak privately with the newcomer prior to the group time and casually determine whether his presence is voluntary; it is inappropriate to make these inquiries during the session itself. Leaders in an open group should be ready to intervene if curious members begin probing a newcomer for her background. The group's ground rules are reviewed in each session. When a newcomer joins an open group, it is useful to emphasize certain rules: that no one is obligated to provide any information or express any feelings he does not wish to share, and that the group does not provide therapy or advice.

People who have been persuaded (coerced, nagged) by family members to attend the group are not in the same category as those referred by professionals. The primary difference is that they are not clearly in the care of a professional. Individuals pressured by their family are in a position to refuse to attend, and if they co-operate and do attend they can still decline to participate actively in the discussion. They may actually find it refreshing to get away from family to a place where they are free not to speak and not to do anything they aren't ready for. If a serious problem does arise, the leader can refer any member to professional help.

6.4 Recruitment and Outreach

Initially, recruitment is essential for the very existence of the group. Without members, a group is one person with an idea. Once the group is up and running and has reached a certain size, survival becomes a lesser incentive. Very few groups become hostile to newcomers; however, once the need for primary recruitment has passed, many groups discontinue or significantly decrease their recruitment efforts.

A warm welcome is not enough. Aggressive efforts need to continue. Recruitment serves not only the needs of the group but also the needs of deafened people. Perhaps better thought of as 'outreach,' this is a duty to the isolated deafened people who haven't heard of the group or had the chance to benefit from it. As indicated by the population numbers in Chapter 1, regardless of how big the group has grown or how long its mailing list, there are always more prospects. Outreach must continue to try to reach them. This is merely persistence with the ideals of the group. If the goal of the group were 'to create a social circle for me,' then recruitment could wind down 'when I have friends.' If the ideals are 'to extend support to deafened adults so they can help themselves in an environment of mutual caring and trust,' then recruitment must continue as long as there are more deaf-ened adults who have not enjoyed these benefits.

For every deafened support group that has existed, word of mouth has been the most effective method of outreach. How-ever, it is noteworthy that membership in these groups repre-sents a minute fraction of deafened people. Word of mouth can be jump-started by sending inquiries to an unrelated mailing list, asking, 'Is anyone out there deafened?' These efforts often locate people who are interested in keeping in touch with the group but not necessarily in joining actively.

Secondary publicity has been achieved through advertising in deaf and hard-of-hearing newspapers and magazines. These still fail to reach the majority of isolated deafened people. Some peo-ple reject these periodicals, but more have simply never heard of them because they are distributed by subscription, not sold on local newsstands. Outreach through medical and professional practitioners has not yet been systematic across the deafened spectrum, although it has been very effective for people with NF-2, who essentially have no choice but to consult a surgeon eventually.

Encouraging anyone to do something because someone else has done it runs directly contrary to the principles of self-help. In this vein, a general concern about collaborating with clinics has been that collaboration and sponsorship may become con-fused with (or made conditional on) endorsement. Tongues wag when rumours start that leaders are receiving special financial or other considerations from, for example, cochlear implant ven-dors. If this kind of rumour can provoke controversy even when the group has no involvement with the vendors, imagine the charges of bias that would rapidly be made if the group were collaborating officially. The effectiveness of self-help is dis-rupted by accusations and perceived bias, even when the accu-sations have no basis or cannot be proven.

The emergence of the Internet is a new factor. The opportunity to obtain information at one's own pace and in relative privacy is a godsend for people tentatively opening themselves to cop-ing with a stigmatizing condition. Also, a computer and Internet browser are more accessible than 1–800 information hotlines and more immediately responsive than postal inquiries. As hosts of *The Deafened People Page*, we have been contacted by many deafened adults with no connection to established groups, who have found us through their Internet search engine. We hope our website will continue to be a resource for self-help, and a model for self-help groups seeking to post information about their programs and to open themselves to newcomers' contacts.

Model Announcement to Professionals and Agencies

A self-help group for deafened adults will be held at [location]. Sessions will be held [schedule of dates and times]. Sessions are [*closed:* registration is for the whole series; *open:* any deafened adult may attend any session]. Communication access will be provided through [real-time transcription or whatever you are offering]. The group leader [do not give name] is a deafened person [specify whether *trained* and/or *experienced*] in self-help leadership. [Statement clarifying any *fees* you need to collect, e.g., 'There is no charge for the self-help sessions,' 'There is no charge for residents of X County/members of X agency,' 'A facility use fee of $X is requested from those who can afford to pay,' etc.].

Only deafened adults may participate in the sessions, and no observers are permitted. Deafened adults are people who formerly could hear normally or with amplification, but can no longer rely on hearing to comprehend spoken information in settings where most people can do so.

The focus of the self-help group is on personal growth and coping. The group will follow self-help principles and will not provide therapy or individual problem solving. Participants will be guided to follow rules for healthy self-help and promote an environment of confidentiality and trust. Participants must have appropriate boundaries; those requiring therapy or other assistance should be referred to a qualified professional. In consideration for being included in this group, participants must undertake to follow group rules and take responsibility for their own growth and self-help.

Professionals and agencies wishing further information about appropriate referrals may contact [who they should contact, and how, e.g., TTY number with relay service instructions for voice, fax, e-mail]. Deafened people interested in registering should contact [who and how].

This self-help group appreciates the support of [credits for any sponsors, e.g., whoever is paying for the real-time transcription and providing the meeting facility].

Chapter 7

Self-Help Leader's Preparation

7.1 Selecting and Tasking the Leader

The leader is not a social worker or psychologist or other professional. This is a self-help support group, and the leader is one member of the group who is willing to take on the extra responsibility of leading the group, keeping order, and organizing the sessions. The self-help group leader should – foremost – be a member of the group.

The leader needs to:
• Be a member of the group
• Publicize the meeting dates or series registration date
• Arrange for communication access (transcription)
• Determine the time and place of meetings
• Make contacts for referrals in case members need professional help

---

Relationships in the group are equal. The leader is a peer who facilitates and shares. When there is no professional in the capacity of leader, the expertise of the group comes from the combined experiences of all the members. The leader has no authority, or *special* wisdom to impart. She simply facilitates and guides the sharing of the group's expertise. If the leader seeks to be a role model, it should be for the introspection, honesty, and sharing she achieves, and not by the exhaustiveness of her knowledge base, or by attaining some level of proficiency in coping, or by coping in a certain way.

An effective leader is not the ultimate, perfect, most well-adjusted deafened person that ever hit town, or the smoothest leader. The effective leader *works toward* acquiring the skills to follow the rules and facilitate the group procedures. She fosters a climate of friendly co-operation; she trains, co-ordinates, and facilitates the group and its participants without taking responsibility for planning and directing the group and its members. The leader should be able to trade places with any other member in the next series with no change in interpersonal relationships – that is, she should not behave in any way 'superior' to or competitive with any member or with the group as a whole. In fact, we recommend rotating leaders periodically, to reflect the principle that members both give and receive help.

If the leader *is* a deafened professional, he and all members must be clear that he is there as a peer, not a therapist, and that the group is self-help and not group therapy. It may be difficult for a professionally trained deafened person who takes up group leadership to resist pressure from group members to be 'more than' a peer. He must be given a fair share of space for his own self-help, and not expected by group members to always be optimistic, cheerful, strong, well adjusted, and so on.

Leadership and administrative infrastructure are different things. If a professional or agency is willing to provide administrative support, such as take telephone inquiries about joining the group, mail out information for socials and upcoming self-help series, and/or provide the space, equipment, and real-time transcription, the group and the leader can make good use of this assistance. Even the most powerful person in the world has clerical help.

7.2 Publicizing the Group

The leader needs to circulate information about the group to individuals who may want to join and to professionals who may want to refer individuals. For an open group, this means getting the regular meeting times included in 'community calendar' listings; for a closed group, just the organizational or registration sessions are publicized. Many television cable companies and daily or weekly newspapers have community bulletin boards where announcements can be made without charge. Some papers have a disabilities issues columnist. If available in your area, consider sending that person an announcement.

Don't overlook Internet event listings. A service agency or community group may list meetings or post a link to your own meeting announcement page.

7.3 Communication Access

You're arranging a group for people who can't hear. But they can't all sign either, and many can't lipread well. So you must have communication access. The various forms of access were discussed at greater length in Section 4.5, 'Real-Time Transcription.' Group members should feel that at self-help meetings, if nowhere else on earth, they can communicate without barriers. This is essential, critical, *imperative*, *vital* if the group is to become a 'safe place' for sharing. The leader has to surmount the communication access issues that we expect the world to handle for us outside the group.

Options:
- Real-time reporter
- Sign language interpreter
- Typist (QWERTY)
- Volunteers
- Self-typing

For group meetings, the best option is the *real-time reporter*, who is a qualified court reporter (stenographer) with advanced qualifications in real-time reporting (CRR), or who is trying to get this qualification. Many real-time reporters do pro bono work (i.e., they waive their fees for the good of the community) for deafened groups. The local shorthand reporters' or court reporters' association may be ready and able to find you someone. At the national level, these groups are aware of this community need, so you just need to get plugged in with the right people locally. They don't owe it to you, but on the other hand it does them good to give back to the community, so you don't have to feel like a shameless beggar for asking. If you feel awkward making a request like this on a phone call, through the relay service, find an e-mail address or fax number and send a note. You will be able to take your time and organize your thoughts to make your case.

The court reporter will bring the special steno keyboard and computer. He will also bring a monitor to display the text, but it is a big piece of luggage so it is more than likely he will ask you to arrange to obtain one through the facility that is providing the meeting space. The reporter should already know how to hook up the monitor. You need to be there early to make sure your reporter can get in the room and set it up.

If people with low vision may be attending, you should get as large a monitor as you can. In any case, the people with low vision should get first choice of seats.

Experiencing the high quality of communication enabled by real-time reporting can be a very empowering thing for group members because they will be able to request the same service at work or school, and in the community.

A second communication access option is a *sign language interpreter*. This can't suffice alone, as people do not learn to sign as quickly as they lose their ability to hear. However, if you have people in the group who do sign, they will find an interpreter more convenient than real-time text. Others find that having an interpreter present is an opportunity for them to see how interpreting works within a 'safe' environment, in case they are afraid to try it, sight unseen, in the real world.

A third option, the use of a *typist on a regular (QWERTY) computer keyboard*, has become much less desirable since the explosion in good-quality, pro bono, real-time reporting. When the typing is so slow, speakers have to keep their eyes on the screen to avoid talking too fast, and this makes it difficult for them to share their experiences fully. It makes people strive to be brief, as if they realize that verbosity is a lot of work for others and slows down the meeting; or it makes them backtrack and repeat where a word has been omitted.

Volunteer typists who are family or friends of group members should be avoided. The friend or relative is motivated to 'help' out of sympathy or empathy or pity for the deafened person and by extension for the group mates. The dynamics are very complicated. Sometimes, because of the personal involvement, the helper has formed a set of beliefs and would like to share them, if not during the session then during the breaks. Also, because the friend or relative is there, the deafened person is no longer free to share feelings involving the helper or mutual friends and family. For example, the friend or relative's generosity obligates the deafened person to be grateful for the help. This warning not to use volunteer typists may seem harsh, but the reality is that you can almost never see the problem that is coming. If a friend or family member volunteers, say no: blame it on the rules. You'll be saving everyone the awkward consequences.

You may have frustrations with volunteers who are not friends or family. If the 'help' is not very good (slow, mistake-laden typing), it is hard for a group leader to deal with it on a professional level without hurting feelings. One deafened person wrote to us: 'We have really poor services here from an always-available Relay Service operator who is very nice, and I can't bring myself to criticize her, especially since she is a volunteer.' When you rely on volunteer notetakers, personal criticism becomes almost unavoidable. Deafened people can be embarrassed into submission, into accepting unprofessional support services.

Passing a keyboard around is a way around the unavailability of typists, but a lot of people can't type all that fast or well, and some can't see well enough to type, and it is difficult to lead a group when someone else can dominate just by hanging on to the keyboard. There are some new-technology meeting room facilities developed for computer-supported co-operative work where each seat has a keyboard and the chairperson has control of whose keyboard types into the group's shared monitor at any given time. This is a wonderful design, but a deafened self-help group is unlikely to get access to one of these rooms.

It is no good at all to have someone taking notes on paper and/or projection transparencies. Why not just go home and send one another e-mail? (We have not yet seen online deafened self-help that actually reflects these principles and rules.) You want full and honest sharing of your feelings and experiences, not someone else's abbreviation of what they think is important.

Most of the deafened people in support groups will be able to speak for themselves; many will also sign when they speak. This helps the real-time reporter do his work. If you have group members who cannot speak, or who speak unclearly (for instance, due to facial paralysis or being deaf a long time and cut off from their own voice quality), you may need to make special arrangements. Some interpreters and reporters are more skilled than others at understanding unclear speech, and you may need to look for a rarer individual if you have this extra need. If the person can sign clearly, you can use an interpreter to voice for her. If the speech is unclear but can be understood with extra attention, you might arrange your real-time reporter so that she can lipread or otherwise make out what the person is saying, or have a second person there to help relay what she is saying to the reporter. While ensuring communication requires effort and creativity, it is crucial that people feel that they are 'heard' and that they can 'hear' others.

One of the things that generic self-help group guides usually emphasize is the importance of eye contact as a symbol of attentiveness. From their years in the hearing world, leaders and members will be aware of the cultural significance that eye contact has. Clearly, in a group comprised of some lipreaders, some sign readers, and some text readers, making eye contact is the last thing that will ensure effective communication. People may consider making eye contact *after* people have spoken rather than while they are speaking, as a gesture of empathy. Slower readers may not be able to accomplish this, and people should understand that no lack of attentiveness is implied. Most speech in the group is directed at the whole group, so it doesn't matter who the speaker looks at. However, he should avoid reading the real-time display – when speakers do that, awkward, slow, and disjointed speech often results. The speaker should be alert to facial expressions or gestures from the group indicating that the transcription may have gone amiss or a wire come unplugged. When the leader is speaking to one group member – for instance, clarifying a rule or inviting someone to speak in turn – he should face that person anyway, even if the person is looking in the direction of the screen.

7.4 Time and Place

The leader needs to reserve an appropriate place for meetings and reserve this space for the time that meetings will be held. Choosing the meeting time is a chicken-and-egg situation. If you know a little about your potential participants and local customs, you can make an educated guess. If not, you can ask around a bit and then guess. Be prepared to adapt to feedback as time goes on, not only from those who do attend, but from those who can't attend because you picked an inconvenient time or location (for them) the first time around. This is a little bit an exercise in the impossible, but you should do the best you can. The availability of a suitable place and support services is also a big factor. If there are no meeting rooms and court reporters on Thursdays, it doesn't matter if that is the best day for the group members.

A suitable place:
- is large enough
- has provisions for coffee and refreshments
- has a telephone and TTY
- is wheelchair and guide-dog accessible
- is in a central location
- is in a safe area
- is affordable, in terms of space and equipment

A suitable place will have enough space and seats for the group size you expect. Group members should be able to read the monitor from any of the seats (a semicircle may be best). There should be provision for making coffee or setting out other suitable refreshments, a telephone with a TTY (or bring a TTY with you) in case of emergency and for those people who need to call for a ride home, and access for people using wheelchairs and bringing guide dogs. Access includes not only the front door and elevators, but also transit to and from the location and accessible washroom facilities near the meeting place.

The building should be in a reasonably central location. People should not be required to fight rush hour traffic in congested city streets to get to the meeting on time, and there should be access to parking or safe public transport (preferably both). If personal safety is an issue in your community, you should ensure that women and people with limited mobility will not be afraid to attend, especially if meetings end after dark. Preferably, the facility will not charge you for use of the space, and will have – and let you use – necessary equipment, such as video monitors for real-time. It also doesn't hurt to have a well-lit diner or coffee shop nearby for those who like to meet up before the group or adjourn afterwards for extended refreshments.

7.5 Referrals for Help the Group Cannot Provide

Once in a while you will need to refer people for crisis intervention or urgent counselling. For this you will need to have a list of people who can handle group members when those situations arise. The list should include names and addresses of contacts; whether they have a TTY number or otherwise how to contact them (especially in a crisis); how they are paid (e.g., insurance if it is not a universal system where you are); and the kinds of clients they handle. Can they sign with clients? How do they communicate with deaf clients who don't sign? What kinds of problems do they deal with? That is, do they handle marital crises? job problems? addictions? mental illnesses? Put this information in a leader's book (a binder is fine) and bring it to each session.

You can also accumulate in your Leader's Book information about agencies and businesses that serve deafened people in your area. This information can help group members locate vocational rehabilitation counsellors to find a new job, audiologists to prescribe new hearing aids, and technical device dealers to get a new TTY or signalling device. Interpreters and court reporters (or their booking agencies) willing to take booking inquiries from group members can be listed. You can also include the phone, fax, Web, and e-mail addresses for mail order businesses, periodicals, and associations, a bibliography of reference books about deafness, and other resources you and your group mates have come across.

The goal is *not* to become an educator of your peer group members. But if people want to contribute information and flip through the pages of your binder during breaks looking to get information for themselves, this is also self-help. Beware that some people spend much of their time acquiring and disseminating objective, technical, and scientific information as a means to avoid dealing with their feelings. If you let these people set the program for your group, you can look forward to months on end of speeches by doctors, tours of captioning agencies and telephone relay facilities, demonstrations of technical devices, and updates from civil servants on policies in development. In other words, this is *not* self-help. Participants become a passive audience rather than helping themselves. You can't stop people from gossiping and sharing news about this sort of thing on their breaks, and the occasional guest speaker special event (*not* during your self-help group time) is a good way to bring in wary newcomers. Your challenge as the leader is to keep this referral information available but off the table during the self-help sessions.

7.6 Other Useful Material

The leader should have handouts to pass out to group members prior to the first session in a closed series, or to take home after their first encounter with an open group, to help them understand the group's philosophy and approach to self-help. A poster, flipchart (easel), or pre-written blackboard list of the group's ground rules is also good preparation.

The materials in the next chapter will help you prepare handouts for the group.

Chapter 8

Self-Help Rules

The magic of self-help comes from the rules. The rules may seem to limit what can be said in the self-help sessions; the paradox is that they enable people to say more by creating an atmosphere of safety. The secret for lasting success in self-help is to be diplomatically dogmatic and to resist the temptation to tamper with the rules. This chapter provides both the rhyme and the reason for the rules you need to follow to get the most out of self-help.

All members should know the rules and the reasons for them. Some rules may seem unnatural, but experienced self-help participants say they noticed their peculiarities only in the beginning: after a while, they stopped consciously thinking about the rules. Some groups permit some leeway; most don't. We explain the rules briefly here, and the leader can explain them to the group.

The leader should be vigilant about what people are saying and interrupt if necessary to control violations of the rules. Some rules really challenge some people's speech habits, and these people break the rules without meaning to; even so, the rules must be enforced. You could choose to overlook a single, small self-limiting transgression, but the leader must intervene if the speaker starts to violate many rules, or the same rule many times, or to stray off topic.

These are the rules:

1. Honour your feelings.
2. Share what you are comfortable sharing.

3. No probing.
4. No visitors or observers are permitted.
5. Everything in the group stays in the group.
6. No advising or individual problem solving.
7. Speak about yourself – use 'I' statements.
8. Speak for yourself; don't speak for others.
9. No cross-talk.

Each of these rules is explained in the following sections.

8.1 Honour Your Feelings

Feelings, opinions, values, and beliefs cannot be judged right or wrong. People are sometimes similar and sometimes different, and therefore there is no merit to seeking consensus or trying to adopt anyone else's feelings, opinions, values, or beliefs. People must honour their own feelings, but express and act on them only where doing so is not harmful to others, illegal, or contrary to the group rules.

8.2 Share What You Are Comfortable Sharing; Be Honest

Make a commitment to yourself and the group that you will be honest in whatever you share in the group. If there is something you are uncomfortable sharing, keeping it to yourself is abso-lutely fine, but telling the group something other than your hon-est feelings is not fine. If the group suspects that a member is being dishonest, everyone's feelings of safety and trust and com-mitment will suffer.

However, the group process depends on members actively sharing their experiences, feelings, solutions, and results and giving and receiving feedback, hope, and encouragement. This quid pro quo is the very foundation of self-help.

8.3 No Probing

The turn-taking procedure guarantees everyone a share of air time and a chance to share without interruption. Every member can assume that the others will share as much of their feelings and experiences as they wish to share. Because everyone will have a turn to speak at every stage of the group, there is no need for anyone to ask anyone else to answer any questions (other than for clarification). One person's curiosity is not sufficient reason to compel someone else to provide personal information. Even information about how a person became deaf is each member's information to choose whether to share. Probing should also be avoided in social discussions. Without a leader to enforce rules in social conversations, it is the individual member's responsibility and prerogative to decline any inquiries he does not wish to answer.

8.4 No Visitors or Observers Are Permitted

The self-help issue – being deafened – must directly affect every member of the group. Family and partners can have their own self-help sessions if they wish to talk about living with deafened people. Perhaps the two groups could have the occasional joint session.

Note that real-time reporters and interpreters are not 'recording' and 'observing' the proceedings. They should not keep any electronic copies of the transcript, or repeat anything they hear.

> *'My [spouse, partner, parent, child] needs to understand my situation better and I thought it would really help if [he/she] could observe the session. Why is this not allowed?'*
> It should be obvious that people cannot always speak freely in the presence of certain other people. There may be some topics where the partner's presence would make no difference, but the topic is not chosen in advance. The restriction has to apply to all sessions so that the group members feel free to choose and discuss any topic.
> It is unlikely that the significant other (S.O.) will hear how the

group member really feels. Instead, there are four more likely negative consequences of the S.O. observing. *First,* the group member will make no comments at all and hope the other group members bring up all her issues and that the S.O. will somehow comprehend that those issues are relevant to him. *Second,* the group member will chicken out and make comments that suggest there are no issues. *Third,* the group member uses the group as protection to launch an offensive attack on the S.O. Here, the group ends up witnessing a bloody confrontation until the leader is able to intervene.

The *fourth* possible negative outcome is that the S.O. will end up dominating the session. He starts out just sitting there 'all ears.' Then someone (hopefully not the leader!) says, 'Hey Gary, what do you think?' At that point the floodgates open. Next thing you know, Gary is telling the whole group about his wife's experience while she sits there having no choice about what is revealed, and perhaps having feelings superimposed on her that she doesn't have. After that, the S.O. intentionally or unintentionally dominates the session because (a) he can hear and so can pick up on changes of turn-taking faster than those who must wait for the interpreting and captioning, and (b) he isn't delayed by searching through complex feelings about being deaf. Mostly, he is giving descriptive accounts of what his wife deals with. Fundamentally, although you think there is a shared experience, there is no true mutual interest between Gary and the group. The group copes with *deafness;* Gary copes with a *deaf wife.* He can *hear.* The common ground, or why we even ask what he thinks, is the morbid curiosity of wondering how others view us. That is not what the group is for. Judging from the enthusiasm that the family members usually show when someone makes the mistake of offering them the floor, it is obvious that they need their own group. Let's hope they talk about their own feelings when they get there, not just swap stories about things that happen to us.

8.5 Everything in the Group Stays in the Group

There is no recording in any form, officially or unofficially. You do not repeat anything – not a shred – of what anyone tells you in that group once you leave, no matter what, unless it is to prevent someone from injuring himself. A 'duty to warn' clearly arises when someone says he intends to harm an identifiable third party – for instance, when someone declares, 'If I can't have her, nobody will.' In that case, there is an obligation to breach confidentiality and to inform the police and/or the individual at risk. How much risk is enough to warrant violating privacy? A breach of confidentiality in the relationship is not something to be taken lightly. Confidentiality is an expression of trust, and without it participants won't be honest with their support groups, and may even be driven away from the group for fear of being reported. (See the box at the end of this chapter for more information.)

This rule also prohibits two or more group members from discussing group members' comments among themselves outside of the group. One reason is that people could overhear. Another is that our main objective when we discuss other people's feelings is to analyse them, and this jeopardizes trust. When a member realizes that a group mate is willing to engage in problem solving for someone else who is not present, it takes very little to realize that the same might happen to him, and the group is no longer a safe place. We have had painful and/or annoying experiences of discussing 'self-help type' things with group mates only to be prodded into discussing the same information in a group situation. The loss of our trust in our group mates undermined our comfort in the entire group.

Some self-help groups (e.g., incest survivors) actually forbid members to socialize outside the group; others (e.g., recovering alcoholics) expect members to be accessible on a one-to-one basis. We believe there is a wide spectrum of readiness for one-to-one contact within any given group of deafened people. Our compromise principle is that group members absolutely have the right to keep their phone numbers private, and to decline phone calls from group mates at any time. Those who *are* interested in socializing with one another must avoid discussing group matters outside the group. This respects the confidentiality of what others said, and what they themselves said or will say.

Another risk that must be recognized relates to the conflict of roles between the two environments. All of us have felt the pressure to maintain in the group our social role from outside the group, whether that is the charismatic social hero, the assertive leader, or the caring therapist. Participating in the group quickly loses its benefits if we cannot let down the personae we construct to present to the world. It is crucial that members have no special expectations from any individual members of their group. Within the group, all are equal, regardless of how they function in the world outside the group.

8.6 No Group Problem Solving or Advising for Individual Members

This includes invited and uninvited advising, and even answering direct requests for guidance. The group is not a therapy group and does not meet to work collaboratively on one member's problems. Each member works on his or her own problems by listening to other people's feelings and experiences and choosing the relevant parts to guide how he or she will cope.

8.7 Speak about Yourself; Use 'I' Statements

Do not make 'you' statements or 'they' statements. Talk about how you feel, not about what they did or are trying to do or are thinking. Do not make statements like, 'When you lose your hearing, you find that ...' This figure of speech implies general applicability. Just speak about your own experiences. By listening to other people, you will find just how general your experience was. Even though 'You find that ...' is often just a figure of speech, there is a powerful effect when you force yourself to make the same statement saying, 'I found that ...' And if you don't, someone else who 'finds' differently will wonder whether he is alone in how he feels. Using 'I' statements keeps it clear that you realize that others may have different views.

'What if I had the exact same experience as someone else is having now? Why can't I tell them how to handle it?'

Because that was then and this is now, and because you are you and they are they. Even if they are exactly the same age, gender, ethnic and religious background, educational and professional profile, marital status, and so on, and so on, there still may be things that give them a different set of values, so what worked for you may actually do harm to them. The exception is if someone is in direct danger, or suicidal, or in an abusive situation – for those people, you can arrange professional help. But unless you are a trained professional therapist, you don't have the skills to handle those cases alone.

Also, you are in the group to help *you*. You can help other people best by giving them the space to work out their own problems. Describe a similar situation you faced, the factors you considered in deciding how to handle it, what happened, and how you felt about it. Then stop: do not say what anyone else should do.

Within the group roles that people play, there is one role of the helpless, dependent person. This person is in the process of convincing herself that things will never get better and that nothing is going to work: 'What should I do?' She already believes that nothing will work, so you will only frustrate yourself by making suggestions she will reject. Group mates can help best by letting her bottom out and truly feel the depths of her hopelessness. As long as she believes she can depend on others for advice, she has no incentive to get in touch with her own feelings. It may be painful for you to watch, but despair (sadness, fear) may be the first feeling she recognizes. The second emotion may be anger that her group mates have refused her pleas for advice. Just be there for her.

8.8 Speak for Yourself; Don't Speak for Others

Speaking for others can occur in two forms: interpreting, and importing issues from outside the session. Members should not clarify for someone else who is having difficulty being clear. Also, a member who has had a discussion with another member, or former member, outside the group, may *not* bring up this issue in the group: not in highlights or announcements ('Terry just got laid off work so let's all give him our support ...'), or topic suggestions ('Terry wants to talk about job hunting ...'), and certainly not in sharing of feelings ('Terry told me he feels frightened ...'). Even if you don't mention Terry by name, sharing his personal experiences, issues, concerns, and feelings is a violation of his right to decide what to share. Even if no one else realizes it is Terry you are talking about, Terry knows you just shared what he told you 'between friends' and will never trust you again.

8.9 No Cross-Talk

Cross-talk is when people speak back and forth. The intent may be to agree, or disagree, or give supporting information, or answer a question, but it is not permitted. Discussion within the group goes in turns, first in sequence of the seating arrangement, and subsequently one at a time when given the floor.

Cross-talk is prohibited because it is not good for the group, because it gives all the air time to the two or three people involved in a particular exchange. As long as people are not debating the rights and wrongs of a particular feeling or violating any of the other rules, there is nothing unhealthy about two people pursuing a private discussion after the group session if both are interested in doing so. If one is not, then the other should not press to continue the dialogue.

Asking for clarification is not considered cross-talk. A good form for asking for clarification is, 'I'm not sure I understand what you're saying.' Leaders need to be alert for abuse: for instance, 'I don't understand – that doesn't seem rational to me,' or, 'I'm not sure I see any merit to the statement you just made.'

'How does it help people to feel part of this group if I can't respond to what they said to let them know I understand?'
Believe it or not, they are smart enough to figure it out for themselves. If you concentrate on sharing your experiences and feelings, and everyone else does the same, at the end of the session you will realize you shared many of the same feelings and experiences. (You will also realize that you had some different feelings about common experiences.) It is not necessary to say outright, 'Hey, Sherry, I agree with you and I think you are right.' In the open discussion of the topic, after everyone has had a turn, each person has further opportunity to express feelings about what others have said, but the emphasis should be on your feelings about what others said, and not on validating the other person's feelings.

Dealing with the person who threatens harm to self or others

Right here and now, we're disclaiming liability because there are no universal foolproof and legally secure responses to the infinite variety of threats that can arise. What we will try to give you here is some food for thought so that you've considered this rare event before it happens and perhaps you won't end up babbling or speechless by being surprised or unprepared for it.

If you believe that someone is about to harm himself or herself, or someone else, you should mention your concern to the group leader. If you are the group leader and you have this feeling or someone mentions it to you, you should contact the police or someone who is formally qualified in crisis intervention. In many states and provinces, you do not have a legal responsibility unless you are qualified in a human service profession, in which case you should make sure you understand your professional obligations. Nevertheless, out of friendship you may want to take some action to intervene in a serious threat of harm or self-harm. Attempting to counsel this person is not recommended. The support group is not a therapy session, and as a peer-leader you are not a qualified therapist (unless you are also a social worker, psychologist, or similar, in which case you should already know what to do). We do not recommend that you attempt to restrain this person. Possibly, you could be sued for wrongful detention or the like. If the danger is imminent and severe, you should inform the police and give them the information you have that will help them locate the person and intervene.

We've included some sample responses not to suggest that these will definitely prevent suicides, but rather to suggest to you how to stay your role of self-help support group leader and not get sucked into the suicidal person's problem and become her co-dependent.[1] Remember that you may be the leader, but you are not her keeper. If someone succeeds with a suicide, it is not your fault and it is not the group's fault. As the peer-leader of a self-help group, you are only responsible for trying to get her some help, and even then that responsibility may exist only within your own ethics and not in the letter of the law. You are in a group together because you share the circumstances of late deafness. You're not qualified to diagnose and treat her, and you may not even know her last name or her home address and phone number (or even her real first name). You have to accept any deafened person in your group if she is eligible to join and is willing to follow its rules. Yet the people who attend don't have to tell you everything about themselves – only the things they feel ready to share, and choose to share. You can't possibly counsel or treat, let alone 'cure,' someone with a mental health problem like suicidal depression when you have no professional training in a clinical mental health field and only patient-selected snippets of information about her. The group ground rules set the boundaries for the group; don't hesitate to reinforce them. Be ready to refer people for professional help.

If the person makes an outright threat of self-harm during group discussion

You might want to respond with a statement similar to this:

> Kerry, I feel anxious to find out that you would be feeling so badly that you would consider harming yourself. I would miss having

you as a member of our group. In the time since we've been in the group together, I have learned a lot from your struggles and your successes. The group cares about you a great deal, but I think you need more than we can give you to handle the severity of the feelings you just talked about. I would like to think you had some professional help you could turn to tonight, somewhere you can go from here, to get help with the pain you are feeling.

You might call a crisis hotline or the police department, or have a vice-leader make the call, as soon as possible, to get the person some help.

If the statement happens early in the session and Kerry seems inclined to stay, the leader might go around the group and ask the other members to express their feelings about Kerry's statement: Do they want to change topics? Or take a short break? Be careful not to make this the night when we all talk about Kerry's feelings. Do not get into problem solving, and beware the risk that the group could become Kerry's co-dependent, jumping 'how high' when she feels the need for attention. You may not have the ability to differentiate suicidal feelings from a bid for attention.

If the statement happens near the end of the session, or if it was so serious that the ambulance came to take Kerry away, the leader may wish to explicitly ask how people felt about the incident. The leader should remind people that Kerry, like any one of us, is a whole person and that her reasons for feeling as she did were not necessarily brought about by her deafness. Since Kerry has shared her feelings with the entire group in this case, there is no violation of Kerry's confidence, and group members may be disturbed by the event and need to clear the air. The emphasis should not be on amateur psychoanalysis of Kerry, but on how Kerry's statement made each of the other group members feel.

If the threat or warning is made in private discussion rather than during the formal meeting, a call for crisis intervention can be made immediately. If Kerry leaves (or is escorted away) early to get some help, the leader should not share anything with the group that Kerry herself has not shared with the group. An appropriate explanation is that Kerry wasn't ready to continue in the group that night. You should not broadcast 'what happened to Kerry' behind her back. When she is ready, if she wants to share the information, she can. People may be curious, but they also need to see that their confidence is respected and that the group is a safe place. If you explain Kerry's private struggles, people will have reason to be concerned about their own private details.

After something as dramatic as that, it may be worthwhile to remind members of the rule that everything in the group stays there, and is not to be discussed outside the group.

If you think the person is seriously depressed but not in imminent danger to self or others

If the melancholy statement is out of order and not directly responsive to the group discussion topic, the leader can interrupt and restore order. If the statement is in turn and/or pertinent to the topic, but seems to reflect a need for more help than peer-group members are qualified to give, the leader can reiterate the group's boundaries.

You might want to respond to their statements like this:

> Kerry, I am feeling afraid about the feelings you expressed. We agreed that we would not do individual problem solving or therapy for each other because we aren't qualified to counsel each other, and yet the feelings you describe need more of a response. You deserve some help to get through the feelings you're having right now. I'm afraid because I don't want you to think that I or the group members don't care about how you are feeling, but we are not qualified to be advisors or therapists to you. For the good of the group, will you go to see a counsellor? During break or after the session, I can give you some names from the referral list in my Leader's Guide, if that would help.

During the 'comparing notes' portion of the group discussion, other group members might also make supportive comments. For instance, some may feel sad or afraid of the fellow member's expressed melancholy, while others may feel happy to have the support of the group during times of sadness. These kinds of comments reinforce the caring of the group, without engaging in therapy for Kerry.

Chapter 9

Self-Help Session Procedure

Each session should follow a predictable sequence that helps build the atmosphere of trust and safety and enables people to get in touch with their feelings after a day (not to mention the past two weeks) of wrestling with aggravations in the outside world. Following this simple sequence will help you lead an effective self-help session, whether it is a single open session or one in a series of sessions.

Self-Help Session Agenda

Start	Topic selection
Relaxation	Sharing feelings on topic
Tune-up	Comparing notes on topic
Administrivia	Wrap-up and adjournment
Highlights	Informal portion

9.1 Start

(Before starting, check that everyone is wearing a name tag and provide them to those who are not.)

Start on time (and end on time, too). Get their attention (flashing the lights or waving hands, or touching shoulders: remember, they can't hear you). Welcome everyone and announce that the session is beginning.

9.2 Relaxation

Start with a simple relaxation exercise. You may have an exercise that you like and use it at each session, or you may ask different people to explain a relaxation exercise and have everyone follow that one. We like the breathing exercise, because breathing helps us get in touch with our feelings. Instruct everyone simply to close their eyes and take some deep breaths and think of a happy place and feel very relaxed. Become aware of the breath. Breathe slowly and rhythmically. Using your own sense of relaxation as a guide, continue this quiet rhythmic breathing for two or three minutes. When it is time to 'wake up,' touch the next person on the shoulder, and have them touch the next person, and so on, until everyone has their eyes open again.

9.3 Tune-up

Go around the group and have each person briefly express 'what I feel right now.' If this is the first meeting of the group, do this step after the review of the group ground rules so that people understand the procedure of going around in turns and the meaning of 'what I feel.' Feelings are explained in more detail in the box on pages 203–5. People are often confused as to what a 'feeling' is, or used to not thinking about feelings at all. A handout distributed beforehand, or a short explanation during the first session of a series, may be helpful.

9.4 Administrivia

Make any announcements, such as members of a *closed* group who called to regret they could not attend, or news of importance to the group such as a change in location for the next meeting. Avoiding overdoing announcements. The amount of other news of potential interest – upcoming sign language classes, open houses at cochlear implant clinics, guide dog information nights, and so on – can become overwhelming and is not of equal interest to everyone. You might want to make a list of the more peripheral community announcements and just inform people where to read this. Otherwise you could get sidetracked into becoming the town crier instead of self-help leader.

9.5 Highlights

Again in turn around the group, ask the members whether they have any highlights they wish to announce. This isn't 'show and tell': people shouldn't feel *obligated* to report. However, if someone arrives in the group some night excited about a new job or a new grandchild, or discouraged about the loss of a job or the end of a relationship, it's good to share that right at the beginning so that group mates can understand the context of someone's feelings. Anything recent enough to be influencing how you feel tonight is a fair item for highlights.

9.6 Rules

Review the rules. If this is an open (drop-in) support group, or the first session of a closed series, explain the meaning of each rule in depth. In closed groups where everyone has already learned the rules, just review the list and be prepared to clarify the rules if asked. Even if the rules have been reviewed a number times, new questions about interpretation may arise. For an explanation of each rule, see Chapter 8, 'Self-Help Rules' (page 183).

9.7 Topic Selection

A suitable topic will complete this sentence: 'How I feel about [...] and cope with [...] now that I am a deafened person.' Each member of the group should be invited to suggest a topic that is of interest to them on that day. List the suggestions on a blackboard or flipchart so that everyone can see them when they are voting. (If you don't have a blackboard, you can write suggestions on a piece of paper and then read them back to the real-time reporter so that they show up on the display. Make sure all the suggestions are still displayed when people are voting.

Don't continue to talk or the transcript will roll the list off the screen. When the entire group has had a chance to suggest topics, ask for a show of hands of people who support each one.

Examples of Topics
How I feel and cope as a deafened person with:
- conversations with preschool children
- being spoken to by casual acquaintances in the locker room
- business trips to conferences of strangers
- when someone says, 'Hey, are you deaf or something?'
- shopping when you can't just use a credit card and have to know the right amount of cash to pay
- friends who don't believe you really can't hear them

One topic will receive the most votes, but before you proceed to use that topic, ask the group if any member feels unable to have that topic discussed. There is no guarantee that every person will be thrilled to bits with every topic the group selects, and nobody has to speak about any topic. Every person needs to feel at least neutral. Some topics may cause pain for someone just to see other people discussing them. The power of veto is intended to prevent that kind of suffering. For instance, a newly widowed person or a person recently dumped in a relationship may still be unready to participate in a topic about 'how I feel and cope with having to depend on my spouse to help me understand people at hearing parties' or 'how I chat in the bedroom.' You wouldn't want anyone to use this veto power frivolously just because the topic is boring or they are not ready to reveal their personal feelings about it. In those cases, for the good of the group, people can just pass on giving their opinions or give brief opinions. The use of the veto when necessary is a very important expression of personal boundaries.

The role of the leader as facilitator is important in topic selection. There is no reason why she cannot suggest a topic (and she should if no one else does). She should feel free to vote on the preferred topic. She should help the group reach a consensus on the topic – offering compromises on wording, narrowing or broadening the topic as appropriate, ensuring there are no members are uncomfortable – so that the group does not lose a great deal of valuable discussion time trying to decide what to talk about.

9.8 Sharing Feelings on Topic

Ask if anyone would like to start. The leader should be prepared to go first if no one else offers. Go in the direction of your choice from whoever starts. Take turns. Go around the group in a predetermined order, such as clockwise. If someone does not want to speak when it is their turn, they may pass. People should feel absolutely free to say nothing, either because they aren't ready to reveal their feelings or because they are still sorting out their feelings when their turn comes around. When others are sharing, the leader should pay attention for violations of the rules, and intervene if violations jeopardize the good of the group. This is the only reason the leader may interrupt, and no other members may interrupt.

The leader must be consistent in reinforcing rules, because if you stop one person but allow someone else to break a rule, there could be resentment. The more freely you give gentle reminders, the less each seems a reprimand. When reminding a member of a rule, the leader must take care not to make judgmental statements like 'you should.' You are calling attention to behaviour, not a personal failing, and should try to emphasize that in your interruption: 'Jerry, our ground rules require us to talk about ourselves and not others. Can you tell us how you feel using "I" statements instead of "you" statements or "they" statements?'

Members should listen to one another from the perspective of how similar or different each speaker's feelings and experiences are to their own.

Once everyone has had a turn in order, those who passed have a second chance to say something. If there are several, invite them to take their turns (in the same order as their original turns, so that no one else has to wonder who is next).

9.9 Comparing Notes on a Topic

Once everyone who wants to speak has had a turn, the discussion is opened to anyone to make further remarks on the same topic. These remarks can be responsive to the comments made in the first round, such as 'I relate to what Harry said about feeling ...,' or 'I was interested that Barry felt that way because it has never affected me that way, but I wonder if it might if ...' There is no need to reach any consensus on feelings about the topic; indeed, it is highly unlikely that all members will feel the same way. Members should keep in mind that sometimes people are similar and sometimes they are different.

The leader must be careful to keep order in this stage so that the discussion does not become a debate or question-and-answer session between two members, and so that no individual member takes too many turns while others still want to speak. Watch carefully for transgressions of the rules, such as 'you' statements, cross-talk, and advising. Do not feel awkward about stopping inappropriate statements or dominant individuals. You can just say, 'Mary, I need to remind you about the rule of no cross-talk. Within our ground rules, we don't get into back-and-forth discussions,' or 'Barry, I'm going to ask you to hold your next thoughts until a few other members have shared what they want to say.' If anyone is argumentative, just rely on a convenient standby: 'For the good of the group ...'

This open discussion ends when time runs out. From our experience, a good duration for the whole session to this point is fifty to sixty minutes, perhaps longer (but set the length in advance) if the group is large. If the group runs out of comments before time ends, the leader can double-check whether there is anything else anyone wants to say. If the answer is negative, you can make an appropriate wind-up comment about how good the discussion was, how surprisingly deep the feelings were, or how much common feeling there appears to be.

9.10 Wrap Up and Adjourn to the Informal Portion of the Meeting

If this is the last session of a series of group meetings, you will now thank all members of the group for participating and let they know how they can find out about the next series, if there is going to be another one. Then invite them to go around the group in turn to say goodbye and share 'how I feel now as I leave this series.' Many of the members will be planning to return; but some will not, and some new members will be joining, and there may be a new leader, so the exact same group may well never exist again. For that reason, many people will want to pay their respects to the group.Once this is all done, declare the session and the series closed, and stand up. If there is the usual (or some special) coffee and refreshments, tell the members where to find it. People can then hug, chat, stay (within the time allowed by the landlord!), or adjourn to a coffee shop.

If this is the middle of a series or just an open session, go in turns and share 'how I feel right now.' Once everyone has had a turn, remind them when the next meeting is (even if it is the obvious 'two weeks from tonight'), and tell them where the coffee is, and perhaps tell them where to read the materials you mentioned in your announcements (e.g., advertisement for sign language lessons, a deaf social event). Then declare the self-help session closed and the informal hour open.

9.11 Informal Portion of the Meeting

After the self-help program, the 'informal portion' begins. Note that you should still maintain the rule about participation eligibility and *not* throw the doors open to spouses and friends (who may be lurking in the hallway). If the hearing partners join at this point, it will stifle some people from speaking freely and interfere with the bonding of the group members as equals and supports for one another.

It is not obligatory for anyone to remain for the entire formal 'hour'; the hour is scheduled to enable the participation of those members who may face practical external restrictions. For instance, controlling partners might deny a member the opportunity to be out for optional 'socializing'; calling the second hour part of the group's time gives the member the flexibility to stay in the safe environment a little longer. Remember, however, that the real-time transcription ends with the wrap-up, and that all interaction after that is improvised. By this point, everyone is well aware that no one is sitting in judgment of any communication struggles, so this improvised communication is often quite successful. Besides lipreading and co-operative clear speech patterns, and fingerspelling and co-operative slow signing, some participants will likely bring out notepads and pencils, or TTYs, or laptop computers.

A great deal of one-on-one sharing takes place immediately after the close of the formal self-help. People tend to approach those who had a similar perspective or experience on a certain issue, and exchange thoughts and seek ideas. While cross-talk is not good for the group, it can be good for the two consenting parties.

If at all possible, the group meeting space itself should be kept 'sacred' and not used for this informal chatting. Even standing around the foyer is better than raising confusion between the safe, special environment of the group and the merely warm and supportive environment of people who understand. After the first session, the group could agree that the informal hour will be held at a nearby coffee shop; the next week, people will park their cars or make their pick-up arrangements accordingly. Or, if they decide to stay in, they might discuss bringing snacks on a pot luck system. (As the sense of affiliation grows, people tend to want to express their affection for the group by bringing food. Self-help brings out the baker in people.)

Because the informal portion is optional, the leader may be afraid that no one will stay; but as the members grow to trust their group mates to understand them, a sense of friendship will develop that will relieve the leader's concerns. If it does not, it may be because these particular participants face long commutes, or restrictive child care arrangements, or difficult working hours, or other circumstances that have nothing to do with their desire to stay for informal socializing. The leader should just keep scheduling the informal time and letting people decide for themselves.

Feelings

The self-help group focuses on feelings, here and now. The past is past, and the future is only partly controllable, but we have total power to allow ourselves to experience the present. During the 'tune-up,' we exercise our ability to pull our emotions out of our physical feelings. During the topic sharing, we go from events back to the feelings we had about them. The tune-up exercise helps us connect with our *feelings* and not just the *thoughts* we had about those events, and the activity of verbalizing the feelings primes us not just to detect and perceive our feelings but to express them. During the wrap-up we again go back to our physical, here-and-now feelings, to put the remembered events away again.

There are no right or wrong feelings. Feelings just *are*. Judging of feelings is not appropriate, either during or outside the group. Feelings do not need to 'make sense.' Different people can have different – even opposite – feelings about identical experiences, even if they think of themselves as similar in many ways.

The first step in understanding our feelings is to feel our physical sensations. Clenched teeth, butterflies in the stomach, knots in the neck and shoulders, or a relaxed feeling all over give us insight into how we are feeling emotionally. The breathing exercise (or other suitable relaxation exercise) helps us get in touch with these physical sensations and understand the emotions that created them. When we are unclear, we can ask ourselves which of the four fundamental emotions we are feeling: *happy, sad, angry*, or *afraid*. Consider these four basic feelings, and then wait for your own emotional state to respond to one or more of them. There are many words to express the different intensities of those feelings – for example, 'delighted' and 'thrilled' or just 'content' instead of 'happy,' and 'furious'

Figure 9.1: Feelings and other forces

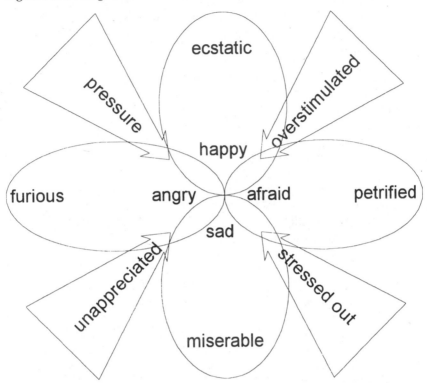

and 'annoyed' for different degrees of anger – and it is highly worthwhile to try to capture that intensity with our language. Figure 9.1 shows *feelings* in oval shapes, with the basic feeling at the core. At the outside, it shows examples of more extreme words within each basic feeling. We can feel combinations of feelings, because we are exposed to many stimuli at any given time, and we have many different values within us.

The arrows in the figure show some of the kinds of forces that we may perceive emotionally. There are many more adjectives in this category. When people ask us how we are feeling, we often respond, 'Oh, I'm keeping busy!' or say we are 'overworked,' or 'stressed out,' or 'taken advantage of.' Those are observations or beliefs – perhaps valid ones – but we benefit most from self-help if we dig into how those observations really make us *feel* emotionally. As a guideline for whether our description of our feeling is just an observation, we can ask ourselves, is this word an intensity variation of happy, sad, angry, or afraid, or is it a description of a situation or forces acting on us?

When we use a term like 'stressed out,' we are stopping the exploration of our feelings before it gets too deep. How does being overworked or exploited make us feel? – perhaps angry or sad. Bear in mind that you do not have the prerogative to compel anyone else to confront those feelings and share them. When they feel that the group is a safe place, and others share their feelings openly, they will do so too, when they are ready.

Chapter 10

Helping Handwriting

Sign language is not the only thing people can do with their hands to alleviate the suffering they experience when they become deaf. While not a substitute for self-help, writing or 'journaling' can provide benefits as well. Many deafened people, including us, have found it healing to write of their experiences, fears, frustrations, and successes. Ours have appeared in many sidebars throughout this book. In this final chapter, we offer some individual writing exercises to supplement self-help in the adjustment process.

Journal writing is a contemporary practice with old origins. It can be a means to preserve history or develop writing skills, or it can be a form of therapy, healing, or problem solving. In this book we are interested in the latter type of journal. A journal brings your thoughts and feelings out from inside, and captures and preserves them so that you can see your progress toward a goal, notice how – and why – your moods cycle up and down, and note your feelings and responses. You can identify patterns, work through problems, heal the past, and map the future. By writing about difficult issues in your journal, you also improve your communication skills. When you are writing, deafness is not a communication barrier for you – you are whole again. Whatever you say to your journal and it says back to you, you can hear it all. When you are trying to determine where you need to go with your adjustment to deafness, you can explore the opportunities and threats in writing, figure out where you need more information, and plan how you will learn more that you need to know. The discipline of journaling provides momentum for you to keep progressing with your adjustment rather than languishing in setbacks.

One perspective of healing through writing suggests that the journal is a place to express your suppressed pain and get it off your chest. However, unloading the pain of the past is fruitless if it is merely whining. It is important to examine events from all angles and place them in perspective. Journaling must involve acknowledging events. Refusing to acknowledge traumatic events may have aggravated our suffering. Journaling also helps by respecting the intuitive and emotional aspects of our experience that go beyond the straightforward facts we process in our heads. The time taken for journaling slows us down, and tempers our pace of living and feeling, and makes more time available for processing our pain.

There are cognitive explanations as well. Traumas produce effects, reactions, feelings, and responses on many levels, both conscious and unconscious. We may be unable to fully understand our experiences and feelings if they remain splintered and diffuse. Our cognitive capacity for active information processing is limited to a few bits of information at a time. Journaling converts a trauma into a story, and we are able to store and process stories more readily because the parts are integrated into a single unit.

Research into the health benefits of journaling suggests that genuine relief is possible. In people with a history of asthma and rheumatoid arthritis, several weeks of writing about their most stressful experiences reduced the physical symptoms of those diseases. Among people assigned to do supervised writing, 47 per cent showed clinically relevant improvement; only 24 per cent of the control group improved (both groups received the same standard medical care).[1] Relief of symptoms was achieved by following a supervised writing regimen, in which the participants wrote about their most stressful life event, which in most cases was not the disease itself. Writing about these events – such as the death of a loved one, or relationship problems, or involvement in a catastrophe – often visibly upset the research participants; but improvement in asthma symptoms was noted in as little as two weeks. Rheumatoid arthritis required four months for improvement to become apparent. The mechanism of this clinical improvement is not clear, nor is its persistence, but the findings suggest that journaling is worth trying.

We must declare that writing essays has never brought about any improvement in our hearing; on the other hand, it has probably played a major role in our progression through the stages of adjustment, and has helped us maintain our mental health as we cope with deafness. Obviously, journaling won't make your deafness go away, and it may not even make your anger, frustration, or depression go away. It may make you feel worse at first, because you will be recruiting painful memories and digging up a lot of buried business. If you believe you may be suffering from post-traumatic stress disorder or clinical depression, it would be wise to consult a psychotherapist and journal under professional supervision.

The other perspective of healing journaling involves focusing on positive insights – moving the positives into the centre of awareness. Oprah Winfrey's syndicated American television program has a broad reach, and journaling is one of the self-improvement measures she has promoted. The aim of Oprah's Gratitude Journal program is to nurture an attitude of gratitude as a means for directing oneself to a more abundant, more positive, more fulfilling life.

> If you focus on what you have, you'll end up having more. If you focus on what you lack, you will never have enough. That is a guarantee. I'm hoping you will learn to take this into your heart as I have and do as we are doing today. We are celebrating gratitude and really trying to inspire a shift in consciousness in this country. And the shift in the country comes with each one of you who hears me today, a different way of looking at your life, being thankful for what you have and you will always end up having more. If you concentrate on what you don't have, you will never, ever have enough.[2]

Use any type of journal you prefer to share five things with yourself that you are thankful for in that day. Everything is significant.
In your daily affirmation, you'll begin to see how little moments
are really big moments. You'll begin to develop an awareness of
your life, which will illuminate life's many gifts to you. Then, the
abundance of life will be yours.[3]

In the gratitude journal approach, we reframe the events of
our life in terms of their positive aspects. When you write to
yourself about your feelings in a nurturing way, you become
coach and cheerleader instead of critic. When your pain is genuine, pretending not to notice the trauma is unrealistic and
possibly harmful. Your goal in journaling is to cultivate the
insight that no matter what the stress, things eventually do
work out in the end. Things not perfectly good are also not perfectly bad. If an improvement in Sense of Coherence is possible, it likely requires this perspective.

10.1 Sitting Down to Write

You must decide what to write on. Many people say that this
most trivial of choices is of great importance. Write on what
makes you want to write. It may be a keyboard, a legal pad, a
spiral notebook, or a bound composition book. The rough paper
of the sketchpad loved by one person could, to someone else, be
an invisible force pushing against the pen. A journal to be carried everywhere for spontaneous input needs to be portable.
One kept for scheduled, once-a-day reflection could be on your
hard drive. Thus, one person's reasoning might be: *I need the
smooth paper for the right feel, bound pages for forced continuity so I
can see my progress and not censor my past feelings, durable cover so I
can carry it with me, and write in it during short breaks in my day, not
too thick or it will weigh me down, pages big enough so I am not
always squeezing one last line in on the page every twenty lines.*
Another person might think: *I need to journal in my word processor
because seeing my messy writing and spelling mistakes inhibit me. I*

like being able to password-protect the document and not worry some-
one will read it. I can never journal during the day anyway and I like
to journal on the keyboard, secluded in my home study, where I can set
aside time for me. If you don't have an old favourite, experiment
and explore.

The same goes for pens: fine, extra-fine, fountain, or felt. If the
pen feels like it's pushing against you, slowing your writing,
then it's inhibiting you. Try another type.

You may prefer to write at a certain time of day. You will need
to be private in the sense that you are able to write without interruption. For some people that will mean the isolation of a private room, for others, the 'detached connectedness' of being
alone in a bustling public place. You may feel more inspired in
front of a window with a serene view, or you may be distracted
by that view. You may feel relaxed in front of the fire, or you
may fall asleep.

Factors that are important to some people will be of no
importance to another. One of us likes to write in a
McDonald's. The pen is unimportant, and is usually a free
hotel ballpoint; the paper of choice is a bound hardcover labo-
ratory book. The other sometimes journals on a keyboard and
sometimes on paper, but prefers to write in private, and especially after finishing a run.

10.2 Online Journaling

Through online diaries and journals, personal web pages, listservs, and newsgroups, people can share their feelings and
experiences with others.[4]

There are websites[5] that provide either open-access or secure
diary pages to participants. (The price of admission may be
exposure to site advertisers while entering journal content or
browsing others' entries.) Many people are entitled to a small
amount of web space through their paid Internet service. There
are also 'web rings' that link many individual journals together:
these enable you to find other people interested in online
journaling, and lead other interested people to your web page
journal.[6]

Online Journaling Tips
- Privacy: Do you want your family and friends to know it exists and where it is?
- Confidentiality: Do you want readers to be able to identify your family and friends?
- Safety: How much of your day-to-day life do you want known by a weirdo who might decide to stalk you?
- Impression: Are you interested in exposing all of everything, or will you hold back the things that make you feel weak and foolish when you think of others reading them? If you will self-censor, consider a more private forum.

Either option provides a means to post journal material on the Internet and receive exposure and feedback. The act of posting is an assertive step that involves expressing aggravations and challenges. You may receive feedback that will validate your feelings about your trials, and words of encouragement to hang on and keep trying. There is always a chance that someone will send insults (flames) or junk mail (spam), but most feedback will be at least legitimate food for thought and at best, highly enjoyable communication.

There are a number of decisions you must make about online journaling. If you are posting openly on the Internet, it is possible that your family and friends will read your posts. You may be able to delay their awareness by just not mentioning them, but they may stumble across them, just as any member of the public can. You could ask them not to read your posts, but there is not much you can do to prevent their reading them anyway. It could be argued that if friends and family ignore your request not to read your postings, they deserve to see what they see. The main concern should be safety – yours and theirs. Many people don't use last names, or use nicknames, or substitute fake names for real names. If you are at risk of abuse, give this the highest priority in deciding whether and how to use online journaling.

It is critical that you protect yourself from known abusers. As many deafened people know, abuse can be emotional, not just physical. If you are in an abusive relationship of any sort, do not journal in a medium that could be found by a person who could misuse the information – for example, use it to embarrass or coerce you. You also need to protect yourself from those who might retaliate against your opinions with further abuse. If you live with an abuser who might find a floppy disk or handwritten journal, you need to store it securely, perhaps with a trusted friend.

You could exclude everyone by using an online diary site just as your storage medium, not opening the contents to public view. This may be a good solution for people who do not want to have books or disks lying around; unless the interested party is quite expert with computer hacking and snooping, your journal stored at an unpublished online diary is private as long as you clear your computer's cache and temporary files after journaling. This way, all your files are stored on a computer at the web server, far away from you, and displayed only upon entry of your password.

10.3 Journaling Regimen

The asthma and rheumatoid arthritis research suggests that the healing benefit of journaling for deafened people does not even require that the writing address deafness itself. There are many people who are not ready to make emphatic self-declarations of deafness, and especially for them, journaling on other severe experiences may be just as healing, to start with.

Unless you have another journaling formula that you know works for you, try journaling using this recommended regimen.

Regimen
- Write for three days in a row, each week.
- Sit down and write for twenty minutes without interruption.
- Stop after twenty minutes.
- If you use a computer rather than a bound journal, do not revise, just input and save.
- Each day, pick up where you left off, until you have said all you want to say on the topic.
- Describe, give examples, elaborate on the topic, event, or issue.
- Write anything and everything the topic evokes.
- Continue for at least six weeks.

Don't answer the stimulus question like a government form – a name, date, or fact is not an answer. Thoroughly examine the event or issue and its effect on your life – don't just record it like a diary. Many journalers find that an initial layer of anger can be expressed but that persisting on the same topic exhausts the initial emotion and reveals other less prominent feelings that give way to a richer, deeper insight.

When you have said it all, select a new topic and continue. If you run out of topics before you have done this for six to eight weeks, go back to an old topic and consider it anew.

Continue journaling for at least six weeks. Then, if you wish to review your notes, or rework them into an article or a letter or a personal experience web posting, or your magnum opus autobiography, feel free. To suit yourself, add new topics and continue for as many more weeks as your like – or forever.

Journaling Tips
- Feel the wave; never mind logic.
- Breathe.
- Get uninterrupted time and space.
- Record the date each time you start an entry.
- Listen to what your soul wants to say.

- Write about all your emotions for the event/issue. Accept feelings for what they are, whether they are good or 'bad.'
- Explore how the topic relates to other aspects of your life (e.g., relationships).
- Don't worry about spelling or grammar – don't backtrack to revise or clean up. Don't pore over it. Be done and move on.
- Don't judge: it doesn't have to be literate, or even coherent, as long as it is honest and you are challenging yourself to tell yourself the truth.
- Write quickly, especially if you find your mind moving faster than your hand and thoughts pass through your mind that you don't capture in writing.
- Have compassion for yourself. Admit the worst, and also acknowledge the best about yourself.
- Don't push yourself to decide how you feel or what is what. Defer 'closure' until there is nothing else to come out.
- Give up the need to be in control.
- Write for yourself, and keep to yourself.

10.4 Journaling Topics

Read through this list and choose any topic that appeals to you. Feel free to make up a topic if this list inspires you with questions and topics of your own.

- What you would say to your family about what you need from them, if you weren't concerned about hurting them.
- What you would say to your family about what you need from them, if you weren't concerned about being rejected by them.
- Why you don't want to tell this to your family.
- The biggest misconception your family has about you.
- The most stressful experience you ever had in your life.
- The time in your life you felt most alone.
- The one thing in your life now that you cherish the most.
- Something someone else told you that you never thought could be true, but is.

- The one thing in your life that you know you can depend on.
- What 'mistake' do you keep making?
- What is the best advice you ever received? The worst? Did you take it? How do you decide what advice to take?
- The worst any 'friend' has ever treated you.
- You envision yourself feeling 'in control' of your deafness when you can ...
- A time or event when deafness was the hardest – a really unbearable time.
- Write the congratulations that you wish someone would give you.
- What plays on your mental jukebox? How do you feel about it?
- The most embarrassing time or event in your life.
- Do you feel superior to anyone or anything?
- What have you given up?
- The thing you would change about yourself if you could change it.
- The best thing about you. Who do you wish realized it?
- What would you tell the twelve-year-old you?
- The event or situation that you fear the most, but that has never happened.
- The classic story told about you in your family or circle of friends – your personal legend. How does it make you feel when they tell it?
- A great expectation you had that disappointed you in reality.
- What is blocking you from feeling the here and now? Describe exactly the here and now.
- Write the rough notes for a speech you imagine giving to the highest body of government in your land.
- What weird or unreasonable prejudices do you still have?
- Was there ever anything you always wanted to do but never did?
- A prediction you wish you never made.

Our Final Essay

There are a lot of silly reasons for not panicking about losing your hearing: How about the news about the economy? Or your spouse telling you there's another household chore? But in reality, if you are losing your hearing, even the latest word about the eavestroughs can seem like music to your ears.

It's distressing to let go of the reassuring world of sound. It's been with us since we listened to the slosh and gurgle of the womb. It's scary to realize that you don't have access to memory lane with a simple spin of a disc on the jukebox. It's frightening to think of how much we have used listening at work.

It's frustrating to go to a box office and be dumbfounded by distant lips behind the glare of bulletproof glass – the same glass that wipes out the last chance at using any residual hearing we might have. My mother says, 'Just *tell* them you're deaf.' I'm certain they would mentally smirk, and think, 'Thank you for sharing,' and have no idea that what I'm telling them is not to recite seat numbers to me with their pencil in their mouth.

It's hard to lose old habits, like hollering a question to the spouse in the next room, then waiting to be enlightened by the response. Drives them nuts that we remain planted in the rocking chair, while they have to dismount the ladder, or dry their hands, and come running so we can read their lips.

There are lots of reasons to mourn the loss of our hearing. But panic? Deafness is not a life-threatening disorder – at its worst, it is a lifestyle-threatening one. Those of us whose lot is deafness should rejoice that we don't have to contend with physical pain or early death. (Of course, some of us came to deafness through some medical condition with these effects, but many of us are merely aging, or took in a bit too much noise in years gone by, or were struck by illness, or have the genes for progressive hearing loss from our forebears.)

If you find small comfort in this as you struggle to find your passport to the mysterious foreign land of deafness – or indeed wonder if you've lost your luggage – consider how much physical beauty there is in the world. The precision of a Swan Lake corps de ballet, the exhilaration of fireworks, the sizzle of Las Vegas neon, the majesty of a mountain, the scent of pine and campfires. Unwillingly cut off from the blather of the world, we become a bit more philosophical. We discover just how much of a sense of humour we have, as we make up the plots to match the stories we see unfolding around us, in real life and on the screen. We gain confidence by proving how resourceful we are and acquiring new communication skills – lipreading, body language, fingerspelling, signed English, American Sign Language, and even *mind* reading(!).

We live in a time when it can actually be exciting to be deaf. Imagine, only twenty years ago deaf people were just beginning to reclaim obsolete teletype machines to gain access to telephone communication for the first time. Today we can purchase keyboard devices that fold and fit into our pocket or an evening bag, and are compatible with cellular telephones, and with pagers that receive and send (!) text messages. We can shop, purchase tickets, and bank by computer. Deaf people are celebrating their unique history. Lest we think we do not share their heritage because we were not born to it, consider that it is a history of triumph over oppression – a circumstance we often share. Today, that deaf people can 'do anything but hear' has become a rallying cry. The demand for reasonable accommodation, to eliminate specific barriers to access to work and social environments, is no longer considered strident.

We live in a time when deafened people all over the world are starting to say, 'We can deal with it together.'

Notes

1: About Late Deafness

1 Schein & Delk (1974).
2 Read 'loud' in the vernacular sense; to be accurate, read 'sound intensity.' Loudness is a complicated perceptual phenomenon. The normal human ear hears certain frequencies as louder than others: a tone of 50 Hz must be 52 dB loud to be perceived as loud as a 20 dB sound at 1000 Hz. The subjective loudness is taken into account in the design of sound measurement equipment, which uses decibel weighting networks to give readings in dBA. dBA includes a conversion factor for equal-loudness perceptions of normal human hearing. Of course, the non-normal ear hears each frequency according to the loss in that ear. Thus, the audiogram shows the loss in the tested ear compared to a normal ear.
3 This is also relevant to understanding noise exposure and prevention of hearing loss from excess noise. While it is tempting to regard a single-digit increase as small, in fact 3 dB represents a doubling of sound intensity. In many workplace noise exposure standards, at high noise levels an increase of 5 dB requires that permissible exposure be cut in half.
4 Richardson (1998).
5 If you graph the *sound intensity* of the total speech signal on the vertical axis against time plotted horizontally, you end up with an irregular wave zigzagging up and down: it looks a little like the oscilloscope display in the robot's mouth in an old science fiction movie (see Figure a illustrating the sound wave of a hypothetical speech sound). This tells little more than overall loudness. With some advanced signal processing and computing techniques, you can do a 'Fourier transform,' which will separate out the

Figure a: Sound wave (hypothetical) of a single speech sound

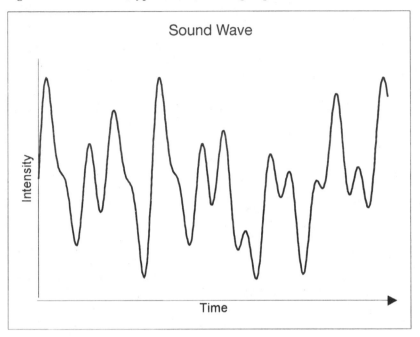

Figure b: Spectral analysis corresponding to the sound wave in Figure a.

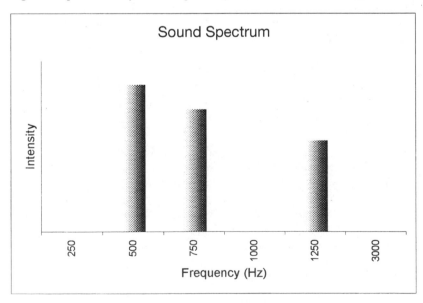

different sine wave components of the complex wave signal (see Figure b illustrating spectral analysis of the same hypothetical sound wave). The sound changes from phoneme to phoneme can be graphed, with *frequency* on the vertical axis against *time* on the horizontal. This shows *intensity* as the darkness of the bands. This creates a *speech spectrogram*.

6 Accents and gender differences change the shape of the vocal tract, but not enough to make one phoneme sound like another.

7 This section is based heavily on Sataloff & Sataloff (1993).

8 Ibid., 188.

9 Woodcock (1991).

10 See Byl (1984).

11 In the medical classification scheme, functional losses include central and emotional/psychological hearing loss. See Sataloff & Sataloff, 1983: 300. These are in the 'functional' category because they are not disorders of the outer, middle, or inner ear, or the nerves. This book will not discuss central hearing loss, a disorder in the language-processing centre of the brain (such as might result from a brain tumour). However, the emotional/psychological type of deafness is relevant to adjustment and support, and warrants brief discussion.

12 American Psychiatric Association (1994), diagnosis code 300.11.

13 Ibid., diagnosis code 300.19. 'With predominantly physical signs and symptoms, or with combined psychological and physical signs and symptoms.'

14 Schein & Delk (1974).

15 Statistics Canada (1998b).

16 Statistics Canada (1998a).

17 Wilson et al. (1999).

18 Heath (1987).

19 Boone & Scherich (1995).

20 Sigelman, Vengroff, & Spanhel (1984).

21 The International Classification of Impairment, Disability and Handicap (ICIDH) was issued in draft form in 1980. The ICIDH–2 (International Classification of Functioning and Disability) was issued in Beta–2 draft form in 1999 for systematic trials in anticipation of publication in 2001. See the WHO website for information on the new classification. Available December 1999: http://www.who.ch/icidh.

22 The ICIDH portrayed impairment → disability → handicap as a progressive continuum of severity; the ICIDH–2 allows either the continuum view or the multidimensional view, the body structure and function, activity, and participation as its axes, and with all three affected to some degree by contextual factors – that is, by environmental factors and personal factors.

While the continuum model is oversimplified, given the different goals people have and the social roles they play, the three dimensions are clearly not orthogonal. However, the new model makes it clearer that people are comprised of many parts; that a deaf person is not merely a set of nonfunctional ears; and that each deaf person's experience can be different due to the state of the other dimensions.

23 Coleman & DePaolo (1991).

24 The ICIDH–2 makes the explicit point that it applies to *all* people and not just to those conventionally considered 'disabled.'

2: Adjustments to Deafness

1 For an extensive discussion of stigma, the reader should consult Erving Goffman (1963). Goffman discussed stigma in the broadest scope, from ethnic and disability stigmas to moral and criminal stigmas. Our observations are an uncanny reflection of those in his book.

2 Ashley (1985).

3 Zola (1984).

4 Spiegel (1999).

5 Coleman & DePaulo (1991).

6 Goffman (1963).

7 A cochlear implant user may still need attachments (microphones, etc.) to hear effectively in some settings, thus, she remains 'stigmatized' by her exceptional tools. Also, an implantee will find herself stigmatized among deaf people. While deaf adults may respect self-determination (but give the implantee a wide berth and a lesser grade of social membership), many outspoken younger deaf people will openly – in deaf college online bulletin boards –refer to implantees as 'robots' and 'freaks.'

8 Zola (1984: 144).

9 For instance, see summaries in Thomas (1984: 35–57).

10 Ibid.

11 Goffman (1963: 13).

12 Ramsdell (1978).

13 Based as they are on 6,857 responses, these results are convincing. Respondents were aged 51 to 61, and held paid employment during the year prior to the survey. 'Hearing impairment' incorporated all levels of severity. Among those with a hearing impairment, 10.7 per cent met the criterion for alcoholism (three or more positive responses to the so-called CAGE diagnostic questions). The rate of alcoholism among respondents with no disabilities was 5.2 per cent. Among those with any

disability, including hearing impairment, it was 7.2 per cent. Consumption of five or more alcoholic drinks per day was reported by 2.4 per cent of those with hearing impairment, 1.3 per cent of those with no disability, and 3.4 per cent of those with any disability. See Zwerling et al. (1996).

14 W., Bill (1976).

15 Jones & Wood (1987); Kyle (1987); Kyle, Jones, & Wood (1985); Orlans (1985).

16 Jones, Kyle, & Wood (1987: 49).

17 Kyle, Jones, & Wood (1985: 125).

18 For example, see Luterman (1999).

19 Kübler-Ross (1969).

20 Kübler-Ross (1995).

21 Robertson (1998: 71–74, 76).

22 Parkes (1972).

23 Cass (1979).

24 Harvey (1995: 3–4)

25 Sataloff, Sataloff, Copeland, & Hirshout (1993).

26 Antonovsky (1987).

27 Cowie, Stewart, & Douglas-Cowie (1987).

28 Cass (1979: 220).

29 Ibid., 220–221.

30 Goffman (1963: 133).

31 Antonovsky (1987: 132).

32 Zola (1984: 143).

33 Orlans (1985: 185).

34 Evans (1986).

35 H. Elliott, cited by Meadows-Orlans (1985: 43).

36 Antonovsky (1987: 106).

37 We refer to this stage as Identity Recognition rather than using Cass's term 'Identity Acceptance' because we believe that the concept of 'acceptance' as applied to deafness is too multidimensional. Indeed, the whole process we are describing here is acceptance.

38 Antonovsky (1987: 142).

39 An essay exemplifying the activism stage was Woolley (1987).

40 Kyle, Jones, & Wood (1985: 125).

41 Indeed, the same might apply to bereaved and terminally ill people as well, unrecognized by Parkes's and Kübler-Ross's models.

42 The concept of 'spread' was described by Wright (1960).

43 Coleman & DePaulo (1991: 71).

3: Effect on Relationships

1 As summarized by Goffman (1963: 16).
2 Coleman & DePaulo (1991).
3 Spiegel (1999).
4 Thomas (1984: 95). Presumably this refers to a speech-range frequency average loss.
5 Entertaining at Glenmont, Edison National Historic Site (1999).
6 Orlans (1987: 104–106). Also, in the newsletter of the Association of Late-Deafened Adults, all five contributors to the 'Letter to My Family' theme (*ALDA News*, 1994) referred to communication as a major obstacle to social support in families. An interesting observation made by Orlans was that members of families with multigenerational deafness, such as hereditary late-onset hearing loss, or couples both having acquired deafness, seemed best adjusted.
7 The latter comment, 'I haven't accepted it,' echoes many comments reported by Orlans (1987: 109–110) in response to a survey of members of Self-Help for Hard of Hearing People Inc. 'I don't think we ever adjust,' 'I am still trying,' and so on.
8 Thomas (1984: 95) reported the comparison of people with hearing loss greater than 70 dB (severe hearing loss) against those who had milder losses.
9 Although the relational aspect of communication has been recognized since the late 1960s, rehabilitation for deafened people has focused almost entirely on restoring access to the message content: lipreading, hearing aids, use of text media, and so on. The concept of relational communication was credited to Watzlawick, Beavin, & Jackson (1967) by Dillard, Solomon, & Palmer (1999).
10 Dillard, Solomon, & Palmer (1999).
11 Villaume et al. (1997).
12 *The Diary and Observations of Thomas Alva Edison*, D.D. Runes, ed. (1968), cited in Orlans (1985: 193).
13 Nakamura (1997).
14 HRH Diana, Princess of Wales (1992).
15 Ashley (1985: 81).
16 Results of a study by von der Leith (1972), cited in Meadows-Orlans (1985: 46).
17 For instance, between urging frank disclosure and never bluffing, Ramsdell (1978) urged deafened people to carefully study a situation beforehand to anticipate vocabulary, thereby maximizing correct lipreading. While practi-

cal, this conveys a little of why the deafened person feels ambivalent about disclosure. The better I cope through preparation, the less weight is placed on my stigma symbols and the more my disclosures are seen as exaggerations.

18 Orlans (1987: 179–180).
19 Goffman (1963: 106–108).
20 Gannon (1981: 422–423).
21 Strassler (1998).
22 Goffman (1963: 134–135).
23 J. Shiels, personal communication.
24 Randle (1954), cited in Heath (1987: 163).
25 Heath (1987: 163).

4: Professional Help

1 Spitzer, Leder, & Giolas (1993).
2 See Fraser (1987: 6). However, Cowie, Stewart, & Douglas-Cowie (1987) reported that only 40 per cent of their sample had seen a social worker.
3 Eight established deaf and deafened social workers and other counsellors responded (fourteen were approached); none reported having received any instruction on late deafness during their professional training.
4 Sataloff, Sataloff, Copeland, & Hirshout (1993: 404–405).
5 Aguayo (1998).
6 Lyxell & Rönnberg (1987).
7 Boothroyd (1994).
8 Also called 'speechreading,' especially by the most ardent proponents.
9 Thomas (1984: 5).
10 Although official objections have, in some cases, been withdrawn, implantation is not *encouraged* by Deaf organizations, and one can still perceive distaste at the grassroots level.
11 Howe (1990: 3, 9).
12 As reported by Fraser (1987: 8).
13 Braddock, Edwards, Hasenberg, Laidley, & Levinson (1999).
14 Aguayo (1998).
15 Janis (1972).
16 The Deaf President Now rally at Gallaudet University culminated in the inauguration of Dr I. King Jordan (himself deafened as a young man) as president. This slogan from his inauguration speech became a rallying cry of Deaf aspirations.
17 For example, Ramsdell (1978) heartily outlined many fine vocations and avocations that might be pursued by deafened people, such as appliance

repair, cabinet making, model building, and clerical services. Admittedly first written prior to the emergence of the knowledge-based economy, this guideline largely excludes any idea of professional aspirations, even in the professional spheres of the day.

18 Aguayo (1998: 71).
19 Sataloff et al., (1993: 404).
20 For an interesting illustrated record of this, see Shroyer & Shroyer (1984).
21 A unique sign-language dictionary that does make this distinction is Costello (1997).
22 Contact signing occurs when a signer feels the other person may not understand him if he uses ASL form. Signing is modified toward a more 'English' form. Signers use ASL signs but mouth the English words. Word order follows the English pattern and uses English prepositions, conjunctions (AND, BUT), and features of English grammar. Signers add fingerspelled words that would be omitted in ASL, such as IS, OF, SO, and WELL. However, mouthing of English words, for example, does not include affixes showing plurals or tense. Use of ASL inflection is also reduced. See Lucas & Valli (1992).
23 http://www.terpsnet.com. Available December 1999.
24 There is a high prevalence of upper-extremity disorders among interpreters that is consistent with the high rate of repetitive motion of the hands and arms. One of the first principles for preventing cumulative trauma disorders is to reduce the amount of motion (frequency, duration, angle, and force). For a given sign, it may be hard to change the amount of force or the positions of the hands and arms, but it may be possible to choose different – or fewer – signs to convey the same message. ASL is more economical in the motions it uses.
25 Baker (1987).
26 Orlans (1985: vii). *Adjustment to Adult Hearing Loss.*
27 Jaques & Patterson (1978). Jaques and Patterson contended that self-help groups have historically 'appeared where professionals could not or did not help' (p. 259), but that the two modalities are complementary and necessary parts of a total rehabilitation system.
28 For instance, see the distribution of references to the website described in Gustafson, McTavish, & Hawkins, et al. (1998).
29 Spiegel (1999).
30 Gustafson, McTavish, & Hawkins (1999).
31 Gustafson, McTavish, Hawkins et al. (1998).
32 Even in diagnoses as curable as breast cancer, self-help networking has been recommended immediately after diagnosis. See Sheikh (1999: 1268).

33 Ibid.

5: Peer Help

1 Deaf people purchase these items at deaf culture festivals, through mail
order firms advertising in deaf newspapers, and through the bookstores
(retail and mail order) of deaf college programs such as Gallaudet University and the Rochester Institute of Technology.

6: Self-Help

1 In fact, fundraising often highlights the 'negative, succumbing' aspects of
disability, in contrast, self-help emphasizes functioning, enhanced quality
of life, hope, and acceptance. See Jaques & Patterson (1978).

8: Self-Help Rules

1 In addiction and dependency terms, a co-dependent is a person an addict
will turn to for an excuse or support or other enabling behaviour so that he
can continue his dysfunctional behaviour.

10: Helping Handwriting

1 Smyth, Stone, Hurewitz, & Kaell (1999).
2 Oprah Winfrey from her syndicated television show episode, 'Gratitude
Day,' which aired originally on 14 April 1997.
3 Available December 1999: http://www.oprah.com/remember_your_spirit/
gratitude.html.
4 While we are aware of listservs related to hearing loss, at the time of writing we know of none that adheres to self-help guidelines. Users must pos-
sess a higher degree of sophistication and stronger boundaries if a listserv
is unmoderated or moderators do not control problem solving and postings
that prescribe The Best Solution. At least personal web pages and online
diaries are more likely to convey the highly personal nature of the posted
experiences.
5 For example, http://www.mydiary.com (available December 1999).
6 For information on web rings, check http://www.webring.com (available
December 1999) or use a search engine to search for individual online
journals.

References

Adams, P.F. & Benson, V. (1991). *Current estimates from the National Health Interview Survey, 1990.* National Center for Health Statistics. Vital Health Statistics 10(181): 82–128.

Aguayo, M. (1998). Rehabilitation for deafened adults: a puzzle with missing pieces. Unpublished master's thesis. Waterloo, Ontario. Wilfrid Laurier University [Available August 2000: www.deafened.org/missingpieces.htm.

Alcoholics Anonymous. (1953). *Twelve steps and twelve traditions.* New York: Alcoholics Anonymous Publishing.

American Psychiatric Association. (1994). *Diagnostic and statistical manual of mental disorders.* 4th ed. Washington DC: Author.

Antonovsky, A. (1987). *Unraveling the mystery of health: How people manage stress and stay well.* San Francisco: Jossey-Bass Publishers.

Ashley, P.K. (1985). Deafness in the Family.' In H. Orlans (Ed.), *Adjustment to adult hearing loss* (pp. 71–82). San Diego: College Hill Press.

Backus, J. (1977). *The Acoustical Foundations of Music.* 2nd ed. New York: W.W. Norton.

Baker, R. (1987). Information Technology: A breakthrough for deaf people. In J.G. Kyle (Ed.), *Adjustment to acquired hearing loss: Analysis, change, and learning* (pp. 80–91). Bristol: Centre for Deaf Studies, University of Bristol.

Boone, S. & Scherich, D. (1995). Characteristics of ALDAns: The ALDA Member Survey. *ALDA News*, p. 1.

Boothroyd, A. (1994). Speech perception by hearing-impaired listeners. *ASA 127th Meeting*, MIT 6–10 June 1994. [Available December 1999: http://sound.media.mit.edu/~dpwe/AUDITORY/asamtgs/asa94mit/5aSP/5 aSP4.html].

Braddock, C.H., Edwards, K.A., Hasenberg, N.M., Laidley, T.L., & Levinson, W. (1999). Informed decision making in outpatient practice. *JAMA* 282: 2313–2320.

Byl, F.M. (1984). Sudden hearing loss: Eight years' experience and suggested prognostic table. *Laryngoscope* 94: 647–661.

Canadian Hearing Society. (1987). *Hearing loss: Questions and answers.* Toronto: Author.

Cass, V.C. (1979). Homosexual identity formation: A theoretical model. *Journal of Homosexuality* 4: 219–235.

Coleman, L.M., & DePaolo, B.M. (1991). Uncovering the human spirit: Moving beyond disability and 'missed' communications. In N. Coupland, H. Giles, & J.M. Wiemann (Eds.), *'Miscommunication' and problematic talk.* pp. 61–84. Newbury Park, CA: Sage Publications.

Costello, E. (1997). *Random House Webster's American Sign Language dictionary.* New York: Random House.

Cowie, R., Stewart, P. & Douglas-Cowie, E. (1987). The experience of becoming deaf. In J.G. Kyle (Ed.), *Adjustment to acquired hearing loss: analysis, change, and learning* (pp. 140–155) Bristol: Centre for Deaf Studies, University of Bristol.

Dillard, J.P., Solomon, D.H., & Palmer, M.T. (1999). Structuring the concept of relational communication. *Communication monographs* 66: 49–65.

Edison National Historic Site. (1999). http://www.nps.gov/edis/entglen.htm.

Evans, D. (1986). *Learning to be deaf.* Berlin, NY: Mouton De Gruyter.

Fraser, G. (1987). Cochlear implantation: More than just an operation. In J.G. Kyle (Ed.), *Adjustment to acquired hearing loss: analysis, change, and learning.* Bristol: Centre for Deaf Studies, University of Bristol.

Gannon, J.R. (1981). *Deaf heritage: A narrative history of deaf America*, Silver Spring, MD: National Association of the Deaf.

Goffman, E. (1963). *Stigma: Notes on the management of spoiled identity.* New York: Simon and Schuster.

Gustafson, D.H., McTavish, F., Hawkins, R., et al. (1998). Computer support for elderly women with breast cancer. *JAMA* 280: 1305.

– (1999). Computer-based support systems for women with breast cancer. In reply, *JAMA* 281: 1268–1269.

Hadjistavropolous, H.D., Asmundson, G.J.G., & Norton, G.R. (1998). Validation of the coping with health, injuries and problems scale in a chronic pain sample. *Clinical Journal of Pain* 15: 41–49.

Harvey, M.A. (1995). Psychological effects of acquired deafness: A training outline. Unpublished monograph.

Heath, A. (1987). The Deafened: A special group, In J.G. Kyle (Ed.), *Adjustment to acquired hearing loss* (pp. 163–168). Bristol: University of Bristol, Centre for Deaf Studies.

Hosford-Dunn, H. (1986). Auditory function tests. In C.W. Cummings (Ed.), *Otolaryngology: Head and neck surgery* (chapter 149). St. Louis: C.V. Mosby.

House, J.W. (1999). Hearing loss in adults. *Volta Review* 99(5) 161–166.

Howe, M. (1990). From the publisher. *ALDA News* 4(2): 3, 9.

HRH Diana, Princess of Wales. (1992) Foreword. In *Dictionary of British Sign Language/English*. London: Faber and Faber.

ICIDH–2: International Classification of Functioning and Disability. (1999). Beta-2 draft, full version. Geneva: World Health Organization. [Available December 1999: http://www.who.ch/icidh]

Janis, I. (1972). *Victims of groupthink: A psychological study of foreign policy decisions and fiascos.* Boston: Houghton Mifflin.

Jaques, M.E., & Patterson, K.M. (1978). The self-help group model: A review. In R.P. Marinelli, & A.E. Dell Orto. (Eds.) *The psychological and social impact of physical disability* (pp. 252–262). New York: Springer Publishing.

Jones, L., Kyle, J., & Wood, P. (1987). *Words apart: Losing your hearing as an adult.* London: Tavistock Publications.

Kisor, H. (1990). *What's that pig outdoors? A memoir of deafness.* New York: Hill and Wang.

Kübler-Ross, E. (1995). *Death Is of Vital Importance.* Barrytown, NY: Station Hill Press.

– (1969). *On Death and Dying.* New York: Macmillan.

Kyle, J.G. (Ed.). (1987). *Adjustment to acquired hearing loss: Analysis, change, and learning.* Bristol: Centre for Deaf Studies, University of Bristol.

Kyle, J.G., Jones, L.G., & Wood, P.L. (1985). Adjustment to acquired hearing loss: a working model. In H. Orlans (Ed.) *Adjustment to adult hearing loss* pp. 119–138. San Diego: College Hill Press.

Language and culture. (1998). Washington, DC: Gallaudet University. [Available December 1999: http://www.gallaudet.edu/~aslweb].

Letter to my family. (1994). *ALDA News.* 8(3): 3–7.

Levitt, H., & Bakke, M.H. (1995). A rehabilitation engineering research center on hearing enhancement and assistive devices. *Technology and Disability* 4: 87–105.

Lucas, C., & Valli, C. (1992). *Language contact in the American Deaf community.* San Diego: Academic Press.

Luterman, D. (1999). Emotional aspects of hearing loss. *Volta Review* 99(5): 75–83.

Lyxell, B., & Rönnberg, J. (1987). Necessary cognitive determinants for speechreading skills. In J.G. Kyle (Ed.), *Adjustment to acquired hearing loss: Analysis, change, and learning* (pp. 48–54). Bristol: Centre for Deaf Studies, University of Bristol.

Meadows-Orlans, K.P. (1985). Social and psychological effects of hearing loss in adulthood: a literature review. In H. Orlans (Ed.), *Adjustment to adult hearing loss* (pp. 35–57). San Diego: College Hill Press.

Nakamura, K. (1997). About ASL. *Deaf Reference Library* (website) [Available December 1999: http://www.deaflibrary.org/asl.html].

Oprah.com. Gratitude. [Available December 1999: http://www.oprah.com/remember_your_spirit/gratitude.html].

Orlans, H. (1985). Reflections on adult hearing loss. In H. Orlans (Ed.), *Adjustment to adult hearing loss* (pp. 179–194). San Diego: College Hill Press.

– (1987). 'Sociable and solitary responses to adult hearing loss. In J.G. Kyle (Ed.), *Adjustment to acquired hearing loss* (pp. 95–112). Bristol: University of Bristol, Centre for Deaf Studies.

– (Ed.). (1985). *Adjustment to adult hearing loss*. San Diego: College Hill Press.

Parkes, C.M. (1972). *Bereavement: Studies of grief in adult life*. New York: International Universities Press.

Ramsdell, D.A. (1978). The psychology of the hard-of-hearing and the deafened adult. In H. Davis & S.R. Silverman (Eds.), *Hearing and deafness*, 4th ed. (pp. 499–510). New York: Holt Rinehart and Winston.

Richardson, K. (1998). Acoustics and speech perception. [Posted 6 August 1998, Available December 1999: http://psychlab1.hanover.edu/Richardson/sld003.htm]

Robertson, H. (1998). Dead wrong. *Elm Street*, September, pp. 71–74.

Sataloff, R.T., & Sataloff, J. (1993). *Occupational Hearing Loss*. 2nd ed. New York: Marcel Dekker.

Sataloff, R.T., Sataloff, J., Copeland, C., & Hirshout, D.S. (1993). Hearing loss: Handicap and rehabilitation. In: Sataloff & Sataloff (1993), p. 399

Sheikh, K. (1999). Computer-based support systems for women with breast cancer. *JAMA* 281: 1268.

Schein, J., & Delk, M. (1974). *The deaf population of the United States*. Silver Spring, MD: National Association of the Deaf.

Shroyer, E.H., & Shroyer, S.P. (1984). *Signs across America: A look at regional differences in American sign language*. Washington, DC: Gallaudet College Press.

Sigelman, C.K., Vengroff, L.P., & Spanhel, C.L. (1984). Disability and the concept of life functions. In R.P. Marinelli & A.E. Dell Orto (Eds.), *The psychological and social impact of physical disability* (pp. 3–13). New York: Springer Publishing.

Smyth, J.M., Stone, A.A., Hurewitz, A. & Kaell, A. (1999). Effects of writing about stressful experiences on symptom reduction in patients with asthma or rheumatoid artritis: A randomized trial: *JAMA* 281: 1304–1309.

Sneed, S., & Joss, D. (1999). Deafness and hearing loss: A global health problem. *Work* 12: 93–101.

References 233

Spiegel, D. (1999). Healing words: Emotional expression and disease outcome. *JAMA* 281: 1328–1329.

Spitzer, J.B., Leder, S.B., & Giolas, T.G. (1993). *Rehabilitation in late-deafened adults: A modular program model.* St. Louis: Mosby-Year Book.

Statistics Canada (1998a) *Canadian dimensions: Population, population density, births and deaths for selected countries, 1993.* [Available December 1999: http://www.statcan.ca/english/Pgdb/People/Population/demo01.htm.].

– *Canadian statistics: Population, Canada, the provinces and territories.* (1998b). [Available December 1999: http://www.statcan.ca/english/Pgdb/People/Population/demo02.htm].

Strassler, B. (Ed.). (1998). *Deaf Digest,* 18 January 1998. [Current issue: http://www.deafdigest.org].

Thomas, A.J. (1984). *Acquired hearing loss: Psychological and psychosocial implications.* London: Academic Press.

Villaume, W.A., Brown, M.H., Darling, R., et al. (1997). Presbycusis and conversation: Elderly interactants adjusting to multiple hearing losses. *Research on Language and Social Interaction* 30: 235–262.

W., Bill. (1976). *Alcoholics Anonymous: The story of how many thousands of men and women have recovered from alcoholism,* 3d ed. New York: Alcoholics Anonymous World Services.

Watzlawick, P., Beavin, J.H., & Jackson, D.D. (1967). *Pragmatics of human communication.* New York: W.W. Norton.

Wilson, D.H., Walsh, P.G., Sanchez, L., Davis, A.C., Taylor, A.W., Tucker, G. & Meagher, I. (1999). The epidemiology of hearing impairment in an Australian adult population. *International Epidemiological Association* 28: 247–252.

Woodcock, K. (1988). Accessibility for the hearing impaired in a community hospital. In F. Poirier (Ed.), *Ergonomics and Rehabilitation* (pp. 157–169). Québec, QC: Les Presses de l'Université de Laval.

– (1991). All roads lead to ALDA. *1991 ALDA Reader* (pp. 23–24). Fairfax, VA: Association of Late-Deafened Adults.

Woolley, M. (1987). Acquired hearing loss: acquired oppression. In J.G. Kyle (Ed.), *Adjustment to acquired hearing loss: Analysis, change, and learning* (pp. 169–175). Bristol: Centre for Deaf Studies, University of Bristol.

Wright, B.A. (1960). *Physical disability: A psychosocial approach.* New York: Harper and Row.

Zola, I.K. (1984). Communication barriers between 'the Able-bodied' and 'the Handicapped.' In R.P. Marinelli & A.E. Dell Orto (Eds.), *The psychological and social impact of physical disability* (pp. 139–147). New York: Springer Publishing.

Zwerling, C., Sprince, N.L., Wallace, R.B., Davis, C.S., Whitten, P.S., & Heeringa, S.G., (1996). Alcohol and occupational injuries among older workers. *Accident Analysis and Prevention* 28: 371–376.

Index

Abuse, 112, 114, 211–12

Accents (foreign speaker), 221n6

Accepting deafness: avoidance, 60; definitions of, 70

Access, communication, 131

Accidents as cause of deafness, 23

Acquired deafness. *See* Deafened; Late deafness; Hearing loss

Activism, 47, 59–60, 63, 87, 117–18, 146

ADARA, 88

Adjustment, 41; endpoint varies, 45; incomplete, 46; model of, 47; speed varies, 44; struggles preoccupying deafened partner, 108

ADL. *See* Aids for daily living

Administrative issues of deafened groups, 143, 153

Adolescents, deafened, 23

Adventitious deafness. *See* Deafened; Late deafness; Hearing loss

Advising in self help, 188–9, 200

Affiliation: in communication, 72; to deafened group strengthened through special interest groups, 150

Age at onset of hearing loss, 22, 24

Agenda for self-help group, 195–203

Age-related hearing loss, 18

Aguayo, Miguel, xii

Aids for daily living, 114

Alcohol, 40, 150. *See also* Alcoholism

Alcoholics Anonymous, 40

Alcoholism, 114, 222–3n13. *See also* Chemical dependency; Substance abuse

ALDA, xii–xiii, 69–70, 88, 121, 130, 147, 151; ALDAcon, 143, 151–2; *ALDA News*, 224n6; Chicago, 89, 129; communication rules, 69–70; founding, 89; original target membership, 89; as substitute family, 69

American Sign Language. *See* Sign language; ASL

Americans with Disabilities Act, 124, 130

Amplification, 94

Anatomy of the ear, 9

Anger, 39, 51, 72, 117

Antibiotics. *See* Ototoxic medication

Antonovsky, Aaron, 44, 56–8

Anxiety, 39–40

Ashley, Jack, 35, 79, 130